Humanity's Spiritual Rebirth

Lessons Lived and Learned from a Pandemic

Forrest Rivers

With Words from Krishna Das

Humanity's Spiritual Rebirth

*Lessons Lived and Learned
from a Pandemic*

Forrest Rivers

With Words from Krishna Das

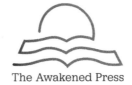

The Awakened Press

For information about special discounts or for bulk purchases, please contact The Awakened Press at books@theawakenedpress.com.

The Awakened Press can bring authors to your live event. For more information or to book an event contact books@theawakenedpress.com or visit our website at www.theawakenedpress.com.

Book editor, Lindsay R.A. Dierking
Cover and book design, Kurt A. Dierking II

"I would like to give a special thanks to Devra Jacobs for being a fantastic literary advisor and agent. Her compassionate guidance cannot be overstated!"
– Forrest Rivers

Printed in the United States of America
First The Awakened Press trade paperback edition

ISBN: 979-8-9912770-9-9

The crisis of the pandemic has forever changed the way we will move through our lives. It has touched all of us in ways that are yet to be understood and integrated into the way we see ourselves and how we live in this world. In this book, Forrest Rivers offers us practices and insights to realign ourselves with this startling new reality. He beckons us to step out of the shadows in our own hearts and move into the sunlight of love, kindness, and compassion.

—Krishna Das
World-renowned Kirtan singer, spiritual teacher, and author of
Chants of a Lifetime: Searching for a Heart of Gold

This book is dedicated to my gurus,
Neem Karoli Baba and Baba Ram Dass,
whose souls reflect the purest essence of the spiritual path.
My heart will always be in eternal gratitude to you both.

CONTENTS

Introduction

When the clock struck midnight on January 1, 2020, marking the start of a new decade, no one could have possibly imagined the utter chaos and unpredictability that would bring in the new year. In March of that year, our world was flipped upside down and our reality of day-to-day life underwent a great metamorphosis. Things that were once inconceivable to us only a short time ago like death and dying during a global pandemic, social distancing, worldwide lockdowns, Zoom™ classrooms, routine mask wearing in public places, and controversial vaccine mandates shifted the metaphorical ground beneath our feet. What may be called a "pandemic consciousness" emerged out of our unique individual and shared experiences of simply navigating life during such a dramatic period. So much has already been written on how that event dramatically altered and upended our lives. However, little has been penned in terms of how our own personal experiences have steadfastly led us on a greater quest for wisdom, truth, and meaning.

Indeed, back at the start of the most recent pandemic when the world headed into the first wave of lockdowns, I began writing a series of articles that described how that event was already helping to grow our awareness. The themes of each of these pieces all approached different angles of that event from the perspective of humanity's conscious evolution. I felt inspired to introduce this perspective because I wanted to balance all the understandable anxiety and fear prevailing then with an uplifting message of positivity and hope. My aim was to show how we could all transcend the minefield of suffering we collectively experienced and use it for our own inner transformation.

As I began discussing the themes of these articles with friends, fellow seekers, and podcast listeners it became obvious to me that these writings would become the chapters in this book. One other thing also became obvious to me: our own unique but shared experiences during that event sparked such a profound period of inner seeking that it was a catalyst for what I now call a "spiritual rebirth."

In my journey to uncover the depths of this soulful revival, I combined my own direct insights with those from the many wonderful souls with whom I had the opportunity to speak. While writing this project, I spoke to numerous people from diverse backgrounds and with highly varied life experiences. Throughout the course of these conversations, I heard many moving stories of personal suffering experienced, epiphanies achieved, and uplifting reflections of how the most recent pandemic added greater depth of meaning to their lives. I asked these two questions of everyone I spoke to:

- Please share a little bit about your own personal experience during the most recent pandemic.
- How did that event add greater depth or meaning to your life?

The gift I have here to offer you is largely a result of the many inspiring conversations I had with all those beautiful beings who were courageous enough to share their answers to these questions. I am eternally grateful to everyone who participated.

May this book uplift you and fill you with purpose.

May this book also serve to remind you that this life is both precious and sacred.

Namaste
Forrest Rivers

ONE

Rewriting the Narrative

ONE **Thursday afternoon** back in March of 2020, I received a sudden email from my college administration that all faculty and students were to pack up their offices and leave campus immediately for the foreseeable future. By this time, the news was starting to circulate that a new novel virus was infecting the world. When I received word of our campus's closure, I recall walking into my friend's faculty office next door and asking him if he really "believed all the hype," surrounding it. Like me, he was skeptical of the media's coverage of this fast-spreading disease and chalked up the world's reaction to misplaced fear and paranoia. Uncertain of how long I would be gone from campus, I packed up my office and assumed that this public health crisis would become just another fleeting story for the media to exploit through sensationalized reporting.

However, in the days that followed my campus's closure, reports started leaking out about high rates of hospitalization and deaths from the virus. I can recall having at least two unnerving conversations with my own sister, Alexis, that signaled to me that the event was indeed more serious than I had initially thought. In those first days of the lockdowns, Alexis, who is an ER doctor in Southern California, began relating stories to me about the utter tragedy she saw unfolding as a medical professional in the emergency room. She described to me heartbreaking images of critically ill people dying on ventilators without their loved one's present, makeshift hospital beds being erected in corridors to keep pace with the influx of patients desperate for medical care, and overworked doctors struggling to determine the correct way to treat such a mysterious new illness.

Like everyone, I adjusted to life in quarantine. And like so many people, I also began to binge-watch the news. I tuned into reports of unprecedented job layoffs and read stories of small business owners being forced to shutter their businesses for good. Not only did this event threaten people's lives, but the fallout from the lockdowns to contain it visited economic ruin for numerous workers who had invested their blood, sweat, and tears into building their livelihoods.

As the lockdowns continued into the summer, the autumn and winter of 2020, I began to hear distressing accounts of a rapidly worsening mental health crisis across the nation due to prolonged periods spent in social isolation. Several of my own students even wrote me emotional emails detailing their own personal struggles in transitioning to virtual classes. They indicated to me that doing so made them feel more alienated and alone than ever before. My advice to them then, as it still is now, was to turn inward and establish a daily routine of self-care with an emphasis on meditation practice. In short, it was crystal clear to me that our society's own fearful reaction to that virus was causing unimaginable pain and suffering for so many people.

As I settled into "lockdown life" I began to inwardly explore a profound question that the mainstream media outlets and our national leaders blindly overlooked. The question is this: Did the most recent pandemic offer us any important teachings in the way of our own spiritual growth? After much self-reflection, my answer is an unequivocal yes.

Despite all the tragedy brought on by that contagion physically, emotionally, mentally, economically, and even politically — it has offered us several valuable teachings that we may point to and say, "Ah yes, that period was certainly a challenging one... But my God, did I learn a lot about myself, humanity, and my own relationship to the greater web of being." In the words of the late and great spiritual teacher, Ram Dass, one day we may regard that experience as the "fierce grace," we needed to shake us out of our unhealthy attachments, egoic habits, and disempowering mindset as a culture.

Personally, I can point to several spiritual lessons that I took away from my own journey during the most recent pandemic. I think many of you will relate to each of these lessons which number nine in all. The nine lessons that we can take away from that event are as follows:

1. Transcending our fear of death helps us live each moment with greater joy and awareness.
2. An "attitude of gratitude" is our spiritual armor in times of suffering.
3. We must live with courage to follow our dreams.
4. Faith, not belief, sustains us on our spiritual journeys.

5. Prayer and meditation have profound healing powers.
6. Forging a covenant with Earth is essential to our spiritual well-being.
7. Creative expression brings us fulfillment, healing, and peace during challenging times.
8. Self-sufficiency is a sure route to self-mastery.
9. Learning to be and to love is one of the greatest lessons that we can take away from any period of crisis.

Each of these profound lessons were offered to us by a once-in-a-lifetime event. And each are the themes of this book to follow. If we can just still our minds and open our hearts, we can hear a counternarrative emerging through all the pervasive fear. This counternarrative of hope can empower and unite us all in one inspiring sweep. Like others who have been inspired by mystical traditions both in the East and in the West, I have long believed that the entire cosmos moves in a perpetual cycle between dark ages (those defined by ego, discord, and contention) and ages of enlightenment in which awareness of our divine nature prevails. From where I am standing, it appears that we are in the opening stages of a planetary shift in consciousness. I believe we are shifting from a dark age to one of enlightenment. If this perspective is given due consideration, then our experience during that challenging time was not some cruel twist of fate or a cosmic "hiccup." Rather, it was something that emerged with purpose to pull us out of our own heartless egotism. Despite the immense suffering left in its wake, I believe that one day in the not-so-distant future it will be regarded as a major catalyst for humanity's spiritual rebirth.

Chapter One Key Takeaways

- The most recent pandemic was a time of profound suffering for much of humanity.

- The suffering that we experienced affected us all physically, emotionally, mentally, economically, and even politically.

- Despite all the real pain and suffering caused by the pandemic, it offered us nine key lessons that are beneficial for our own spiritual growth.

- These nine teachings are as follows: Transcending our fear of death helps us live each moment with greater joy and awareness; an "attitude of gratitude" is our spiritual armor in times of suffering; we must live with courage to follow our dreams; faith, not belief, sustains us on our spiritual path; prayer and meditation have transformative effects on one's own life; forming a covenant with Earth is essential to our well-being; self-sufficiency is a sure route to self-mastery; creative expression brings us fulfillment, healing, and peace during challenging times; learning how to be and to love is the greatest lesson that we can take away from any period of crisis.

- The most recent pandemic played an important role in the planetary shift of consciousness already underway.

Chapter One Meditation

Find a comfortable position seated either upright or with legs crossed. Now close your eyes and tune into your breath. Breathe in and breathe out. As you inhale and exhale, try to recall a difficult situation in your life. That difficult situation could be anything from a romantic breakup to the death of a beloved family member or pet, to enduring a sickness or disease or losing a job. Feel the weight of that pain in your heart and acknowledge the residue of trauma that remains from that event. Note the feelings that you experience as you relive that moment. Are they feelings of sadness? Anger? Confusion? Whatever those feelings, allow them to enter your stream of consciousness for the moment. As you sit with these emotions, gently repeat the following mantra to yourself: "I am not my pain, I am loving awareness." Continue to repeat this mantra to yourself.

After reliving the painful emotions that accompanied this difficult time in your life, now direct your attention to the myriad ways in which this event positively spurred your own spiritual growth. Maybe a new romantic relationship blossomed out of the ending of an old one. Or maybe the death of a loved one made you more appreciative for the impermanence of our time in these forms. Maybe that job you lost wound up giving you the courage to change occupations that are better suited for your spiritual journey. As you continue to contemplate how this trying event benefited your own personal growth, end your meditation by gently repeating this second mantra: "I now transcend my pain through the act of acceptance." Open your eyes and draw three long breaths. In and out.

OM.

TWO
Transcending our Fear of Death

Our Fear of Death as Westerners

OUR **existence in** these forms can be boiled down to two things: birth and death. By some mysterious and mystical process, we take birth in these bodies, we grow old, and then we die. Yet even though both birth and death form the spiritual essence of who we are, so many of us in Western culture embrace the former while recoiling from the latter. It is plainly obvious that we Westerners love the moment of birth. We are filled with joy the first time a newborn opens its eyes. We get high on the love vibes of a newfound romance. And we toast in celebration with friends when we earn that promotion at work or experience the good fortune of realizing a long-held dream. But when it comes down to the moment of saying goodbye to a beloved person or pet, letting go of a broken relationship or acknowledging the passing of our own youth, so many of us withdraw into the deepest recesses of our minds and attempt to deny the other half of our existence. In truth, death is always present. And in truth, death is our greatest teacher. So why do so many Westerners have such an aversion to death?

For one, the intense emotion of grief that comes with loss can simply feel too overwhelming. In my own case, I can still vividly remember my first encounter with death and watching as a thirteen-year-old boy on the night that my grandfather was taken away by ambulance after suffering a major stroke. I recall visiting him in the hospital over the next three days of his recovery and rejoicing over the fact that he had survived. However, as fate would have it, my grandfather suffered a second stroke the fourth day and passed soon after. As a teenager, I couldn't comprehend the loss. Where had he gone? And why did someone that close to me (we lived under the same roof for six years) have to die? The grief I felt in the wake of his passing was so overwhelming that when my grade schoolteachers excused me from a week of classes, I took only two days off to keep myself distracted from the sheer pain I was feeling at the time.

I am sure many of you have experienced this same sense of grief following the passing of a loved one. Grief is among the most painful and profound emotions that a human being can endure. Even the most spiritually evolved being will struggle to keep their heart open to the many soulful lessons that grief bestows upon us. So undoubtably, the fear we feel in having to confront the intense emotions of grief that follows in the wake of death may explain why we have such an aversion to it in the first place. Of course, it doesn't help that here in the West we don't embrace death quite as openly as in cultures like India, where it is more consciously accepted as a natural fact of life.

Another reason why humans (particularly in the West) tend to have such a fear of death is because every encounter we have with it is something of a mini-dress rehearsal for that ultimate of inevitable moments: when we too must die. Somewhere deep within we are aware that each passing of a loved one, each moment of a relationship ending, and each farewell to a passing chapter in our lives is preparing us for the time when we must let go of our bodies. The very thought of having to die and leave loved ones behind can be a lot for people to bear. As we prepare to die, the thought that we may cease to exist at all can also be a source of great anxiety. This fear is particularly acute among avowed atheists or those with agnostic leanings.

Before arriving on the path myself, I used to be one of those people. Before turning on to meditation practice and reading the words of realized saints and sages that left me without a shadow of a doubt that our souls continue after we drop our bodies, I just assumed that when you die, that was it. Plain and simple. I was firm in my belief that who I am is my body. The thought of no longer existing truly terrified me. So much so, that I even convinced myself into thinking I would never die! How far down the road of delusion must I have gone to come to that conclusion! Looking back now, this lack of personal faith in an afterlife prevented me from fully opening to the inevitability of my own death. Not surprisingly, all those "little deaths" I endured along the way, like a breakup or moving, elicited such great discomfort within me that I turned to heavy drinking to partially push away my own fear of dying. I would suspect that deep down, these same existential fears are and have been experienced by countless other beings.

Extreme interpretations of certain religious scriptures also explain why so many Westerners have such a fear of death. As many people who were raised in the church can attest to, certain fundamentalist sects teach that true believers will be rewarded in a crucial moment of ultimate judgment with an eternal afterlife of heaven. On the surface this sounds nice. Who wouldn't want to experience the paradise of eternal heaven? However, for those "non-believers," "sinners," and "pagans," these same interpretations are clear what will meet them after death: eternal hellfire! Such fear-inducing notions as "eternal damnation" do not exactly help one go gently into the night of death. Of course, a word must be said for all those inspiring mystics who have gone far beyond such fundamentalist teachings of the church and forged a direct relationship with the consciousness of Christ to find that God is one of total love and forgiveness. How could an all-loving God ever condemn fractals of its own universal essence to such a fate? No matter how far off some souls may have wandered, does God's omnificent grace not extend to all in the promise of their soul's redemption?

Fear in the Most Recent Pandemic

The fear of death was a constant theme that emerged from the many conversations I had with people. The sheer existential nature of that event compelled many of us to explore those questions that have been put forth to us by the mystics of every faith and religion through the ages. Some of these questions include but are not limited to the following:

- What is death?
- Who or what dies when we drop the body?
- Where do we go after passing on?
- In what ways can the presence of death contribute to our own personal growth?

For some seekers, the most recent pandemic was the first time that they had ever thought about their own mortality. For Jason P., a grocery store worker from Asheville, North Carolina, that event was a "revelation" in terms of his relationship to death. Jason explained:

> For much of my adult life I had never really thought of death. I just assumed that death was something that happened to other people when they were old but not me. But as an "essential worker" during that pandemic, I unknowingly came face to face with several people in the public who were sick, and I knew many co-workers who came down with the virus. Finally, about six months into the pandemic, I contracted it (the virus) myself and that's when I really think I started to ask some deeper questions about death and re-examine my own life. [2]

For Alex C., an environmental engineer and dear friend of mine from Rochester, New York, the contagion also provided him with grist for the mill with which to deepen his own meditation practice on death and dying. Alex, who has practiced Zen meditation for over twelve years, explained that the most recent pandemic helped him delve more deeply into his own practice as well as reflect upon how consciously he was living his own life. In Alex's words:

> Obviously, the pandemic provided fertile ground for me to deeply contemplate death. Death is something that I have always thought about and been aware of ever since I was a child. Without question, I think the pandemic has made me reflect more deeply on my own mortality and of how mindfully and skillfully I am living this life now. [3]

For Erica B., an editor of a fantastic (online) Canadian conscious living publication, the viral epidemic initially brought up some uncomfortable feelings regarding her own mortality:

> I have asthma. So early on at the start of that pandemic I became anxious about getting sick and obviously I did everything I could do to keep myself safe. However, as the pandemic dragged on, I started to reflect more deeply about my predicament and concluded that while I could choose to be careful there was only so much control I had over the situation. In a sense, that event has taught me to let go. It has also taught me to become a bit more comfortable with my own mortality and with the understanding that I could succumb to death at any point. Strangely, this realization has brought me greater peace. [4]

A Useful Practice during a Pandemic

I can relate to the profoundly existential nature of the comments from Jason, Alex, and Erica above. In the summer of 2021, at the height of the virus's spread, I thought it was an appropriate time to take on a personal forty-day challenge to live each day with death on my mind. This challenge was inspired by the late spiritual teacher Stephen Levine in his book, *A Year to Live*, a classic manual for conscious living and dying. In the spirit of Levine, I resolved to keep a "death journal," in which I would offer my daily reflections and meditations on specific themes related to death. During the forty-day period, I partook in the Buddhist Maranasati practice (meditation on one's own death), reflected on my first encounter as a child with it, looked to the natural world for answers about birth and death, and spent many nights in silent contemplation of the future passing of loved ones.

Throughout this forty-day exercise, two intentions were always foremost on my mind. The first was to cultivate greater joy in my life though opening more deeply to each moment. The second was to constantly remember the impermanent nature of our physical reality. Through activities like hiking in nature, I experienced the overflowing joy, unbounded freedom, and mysterious wonder of a child. And through exercises like the Buddhist Maranasati practice and recitation of certain death mantras (inspired by Levine's own death chants), I managed to keep death and dying on my mind for the forty days. In more fully opening to death, I noticed that time seemed to slow down yet somehow each moment grew with greater urgency. This is among the most important lessons I took away from the challenge: each moment is truly sacred and filled with meaning. Knowing that we can die at any moment should be enough for us all to rise from our chairs and live our lives with more passion.

Anyone can do this practice. But be warned: it is not for the faint of heart! During this forty-day period, I experienced greater joy and became more aware of the impermeant nature of my physical body. As an added positive benefit, I also became more identified with the soul plane. Working through my own fears of death and dying allowed me to REALLY see that while our bodies will inevitably die, some eternal essence of who we are (call it the soul or the self) is deathless. I have long believed that our spirits are infinite, but during those forty days this mere belief solidified into a firmer faith.

However, despite all the personal breakthroughs and insights I encountered during those forty days, I also experienced moments when my old fears of death crept back up on me. Two examples stand out. On the fifth day of the challenge, my old publisher, Aaron Y., passed away. Less than one month before dropping his body, Aaron had learned the devastating news that he had stage 4 cancer. His sudden death hit me like a ton of bricks. For days afterward, I asked myself why someone so positive and caring (Aaron was really such a beautiful and kind soul who always believed in me) must suffer through such a painful and sudden death.

I really stewed on this for a long time because something about the nature of his death just didn't sit right with me. So... There I was on an ego trip (yet again) somewhat self-righteously judging events of the universe as if I knew how it should all really go down. And that's when it hit me. We truly have no control over the time and manner of our passing. As the great Indian saint Neem Karoli Baba taught, we don't die one moment before or after we are supposed to. When our time comes to transcend our forms, that is it. There can be no bargaining it away. No holding it off for tomorrow. The wheel of birth and death fatefully turns down the karmic road of creation.

The other moment that really exposed my old fears happened while flying on a plane during the twenty-first day of the challenge. Ever since I was young, I have always had a fear of flying. But flying during a pandemic only seemed to worsen my anxiety. Upon arriving at the Atlanta International Airport that day, I recall feeling more on edge than usual. Seeing everyone wearing face masks was unsettling. It felt like I was trapped in some bad zombie apocalypse movie where my fear of contracting the virus somehow equaled my fear of flying. Of course, as I boarded my flight and settled into my customary seat by the aisle, I felt that familiar fear rising inside me once again.

As the plane took off, I attempted to calm my mind by repeating the Maha Mantra (the Great mantra in the Hindu faith devoted to Sri Krishna). Repeating those sacred words greatly helped ease my discomfort. But then, about an hour into the flight, the plane hit bad turbulence and I felt an anxiety attack coming on. As the turbulence worsened, I noticed that both my forehead and the palms of my hands were covered in sweat and that my breathing had grown fast and shallow. Then something miraculous happened in that moment of sheer terror: I somehow managed to flip into the witness mode for just a minute to see that my fear of death was at the root of all my anxiety. As soon as I acknowledged this fear, I began to instantly calm down and rode through the remaining turbulence with only mild worry. While I ended up working through my fears during the flight, I had still allowed myself to be sucked into my own paranoid melodrama. When the plane safely landed and I exited at my gate, all I could do was laugh at my own irrational fears of dying while flying.

Transcending Our Fear of Death

Of course, a hallmark of any global pandemic is our emphasis on the number of dead and dying. Understandably, the repetition of mounting casualties by the media constantly provoked deep anxiety and fear among the people. However, our experience with death during that time provided us with an important opportunity to confront our own fears of it. But why is it so important for us to confront this intrinsic fear? Because it allows us to live our lives with a greater sense of freedom and equanimity. I strongly believe that making peace with death is among the highest practices we can pursue. When we transcend our own fear of it, we unlock a gate to live more deeply in the present moment. When we can do that, we follow our dharma, our unique karmic path, and all of humanity's benefits.

For seekers like Lisa K., a Pennsylvania school bus driver, the most recent pandemic provided a valuable opportunity to do just that — to transcend the fear of death and work for the healing of humanity:

I did not live in fear of the virus. Looking back now, I have a tremendous amount of disappointment in how many chose to respond in behavior with anger and neglect for one another. I find I'm happiest hanging with my tribe of family and friends now. Transcending my fear of dying has allowed me to spend more time in prayer for the healing of this planet. I have grown more within to seek and manifest great love. I place great emphasis now on finding my peace and happiness with great joy and gratitude for who I am and where I am in my journey on planet Earth. [5]

For Paul G., a bartender from Littleton, Colorado, that event was a difficult time for him personally, but it provided him with an opportunity to let go of a lifelong fear of death:

The pandemic was a really challenging time for me. When the restaurant where I tend bar at was forced to close in March of 2020, I spent six anxious months on unemployment. I knew many friends in the restaurant business who got sick with the virus. Eventually, I caught a bad case of it myself, but I fortunately recovered without any long-term effects. However, during that difficult period of being unemployed and getting sick, I began to spend more time reading spiritual books and practicing meditation for the first time. Most significantly, when it was time to return to work, I found that I had shed my fear of death. I later realized that this fear had hindered my evolution as a human being. I can't begin to describe how thankful I am that I had those six months to do some serious work on myself. Living without the fear of dying has been among the most liberating experiences I have had. [6]

As is clear through Lisa and Pauls' experiences, the most recent pandemic provided a valuable chance to confront our fear of death. That event was a dramatic reminder that one day, sooner or later, we are all going to die. It also taught us that as we draw closer to our own death, we are each presented with two paths that we can follow. We can choose the first and heavily conditioned road of denying the inevitable passing of our bodies and blindly grasp to the fleeting nature of this material world. But this choice will only wind up creating more needless suffering. For just as the Buddha taught, we cannot hold on to any physical forms, including our bodies.

Very fortunately, many of us have discovered that there is a second path we can follow. We always have the choice to embrace our own death by surrendering to the passage of form back to the formless — the Void, or the One. Instead of continually running from death's haunting shadow, we have the power to meet it at its own doorstep with our hearts fully open to what IS and will soon become. Rather than lament the fact that we really have no control over the time and manner of our own passing, we can choose to become death's supreme inquisitor and ask it all the questions that we already intuitively know the answers to. Death does not have to be a painful and frightening process. We can use this ultimate of transitions for our own inner healing and personal growth.

Despite the immense suffering left in its wake, the contagion was our fierce and noble teacher by showing us how to live more fully through transcending our fear of death.

Chapter Two Key Takeaways

- Westerners tend to have an acute fear of death.

- This existential fear is primarily driven by four things: our culture's aversion to death and dying, our conditioned tendency to avoid suffering and the grieving process, a lack of faith in the soul's continuance after death, and extremist interpretations of religious scripture.

- The most recent pandemic presented a valuable opportunity for many to contemplate their own death.

- That event was a profound reminder that the time and manner of our death is outside of our control.

- Knowing that the time and manner of our death is outside our control infuses each moment with an added sense of urgency and meaning.

- Living at least thirty days with death on your mind is an effective spiritual practice to try during a pandemic.

- The process of transcending our fear of death allows us to live with less anxiety and greater equanimity when a dramatic event such as a pandemic does occur.

- Death does not have to be something that we fear. It can be a catalyst for personal healing and growth.

Chapter Two Meditation

Find a comfortable position seated either upright or with legs crossed. Now close your eyes and tune into your breath. Breathe in and breathe out. Try to imagine the moment of your own death. Picture where you are during this most transformative event. Maybe you are at home resting peacefully in bed. Or maybe you are out in nature sitting against a favorite tree or taking in one final sunset at the ocean. Wherever you are, try and recall the sights and smells of the environment you are in. Are the sights and sounds sweet and pleasant? Or are they bitter and unpleasant? Whatever their quality, do not attach yourself to these senses. Simply take note of your environment without casting too much judgment.

Now as you continue to deeply inhale and exhale, try to imagine the people that surround you on your death bed. Maybe your son or daughter (or both) are standing by holding your hand. Or maybe some dear friends and a beloved pet are with you in those final moments as you prepare to drop your body. As your loved ones surround you, try to sense how they are feeling. Are they resonating vibrations of fear and grief for your predicament? Or do the vibrations of unconditional love and total acceptance resonate in the room? As you draw your final breaths, try to imagine what you will say to those loved ones present. Will you tell them you love them? Or will you share any of your life's regrets and issue apologies? Maybe you will simply nod and smile at them in a glowing recognition of that inevitable moment when you take off that tight shoe and become a deathless spirit once again. Now, try to imagine the final seconds just before your passing. What is the final thought on your mind as your soul exits your body? Is it a prayer to Christ, Buddha, or Krishna? Or is your final thought really words of gratitude like, "Thank you Divine Universe," or, "To the formless Void I return"? As you picture drawing your last breath in this form, hold onto your final thought. For this thought, it is believed by various mystics, will determine the circumstances of your soul's journey in its next birth. Slowly open your eyes and repeat this mantra three times:

> "Though my body will die
> My spirit is free
> And I know myself as part
> Of this eternal cycle:
> Birth, Life, Death, Rebirth."

OM.

THREE
The Light of Gratitude

The Power of Gratitude: A Personal Tale

FEW things have the power to totally transform one's life as gratitude. Gratitude is the wellspring of happiness and the foundation of love. It is also the anchor of true faith and genuine humility. Without gratitude, the toxic stew of bitterness, jealousy, and regret boils over inside us. I would know. As a teenager and as a young man, I lived life without gratitude and experienced the terrible pain of doing so. Outwardly, I appeared to be a friendly, happy, and gracious person. I could make any person laugh and I was loyal to my friends through thick and thin. However, beneath the surface an intense fire raged within me. Despite receiving boundless love and attention from my wonderful family, I was inwardly resentful about my adoption as a child. For many years, three bitter questions ran on repeat in my own mind:

- Why did my birth mother give me up for adoption when I was only months old?
- Why did I try so desperately hard to win acceptance from others when it was clear that I just didn't fit in anywhere?
- Why did I have to experience the pain and confusion of not truly belonging?

As I allowed these questions to dominate my thoughts, I began to experience a range of negative and unpleasant emotions as a result. Among the worst of these feelings was that I came to see myself as a victim of circumstance. Of course, as I would later realize, this couldn't have been further from the truth. Far from being a victim of circumstance, I was a blessed recipient of God's grace. But at the time I couldn't see that. Eventually, my sense of resentment about the adoption contributed to destructive behaviors like heavy drinking. Throughout the entirety of my twenties and on into my early thirties I filled my desperate need for belonging with endless partying and a hedonistic lifestyle. During those years, I endured many unhealthy romantic relationships with women, partook in too many wild nights of drinking to count, and I frequently found myself in brushes with police. During that difficult time in my life, I also seriously contemplated committing suicide. Had it not been for the torturous thought of inflicting such an emotional toll on my family, I am quite certain that I would have taken my own life.

My own refusal to put in the long hours on myself and address the adoption led me in a downward spiral. My self-inflicted discontentment continued right up to my thirty-first birthday. And that's when something miraculous happened. While on a vacation in Maui, Hawaii, I experienced an awakening while hiking in the breathtaking beauty of nature. On the third or fourth day of the trip, I was wandering on a little spur trail that led me to the edge of a breathtaking cliff overlooking the crystal blue ocean. In that moment I was so overwhelmed with joy that I instantly tore off all my clothes and let out a great (and naked!) primal yell! Today, when I reflect on what I truly felt in that moment, it was pure gratitude. I felt pure gratitude to be alive. I felt pure gratitude to finally know that I was a part of something infinitely greater than my mind could ever comprehend. While standing there in awe of Earth's wonder, I also felt an overflowing gratitude for my adoption.

Suddenly, everything about my adoption made perfect sense. It was my destiny to be adopted into the family I was in. It was also an incomprehensibly high and selfless act of love for my birth mother to give me up for adoption knowing that I would have more doors opened to me in America. And of course, it was also an incomprehensibly high and selfless act of love for my adopted mother to endure horrific physical abuse and an exhausting legal battle just to get me out of Greece. In that moment I was catapulted into a higher realm of consciousness where the boundary dissolved between who it was that thought they were the knower and the subject they thought was being known. In that moment, there was no me. There was no birth mother. There was no adopted mother and father. We were all just one perfect expression of love. The point of this somewhat long-winded story is that no spiritual breakthrough for me would have even been possible without the power of gratitude. For gratitude was at the root of that profound glimpse of reality I experienced in that indescribably perfect moment.

Giving Thanks During a Pandemic

While writing this book I noticed something very hopeful and inspiring: despite all the doom and gloom narratives in the media's coverage of the most recent pandemic, many people still found reason to express their gratitude during an otherwise difficult time. For many, the period of government-enforced lockdowns proved fertile grounds for the cultivation of greater gratitude. On the one hand, the lockdowns were no doubt unsettling, isolating, and even frightening for countless millions of people. However, on the other hand, they also offered profound and valuable lessons for spiritual growth in the way of gratitude.

For Brett U., an environmental engineer from Charleston, South Carolina, the overall egoism and selfishness on display in response to the virus affected him (in his own words) "like a knife going the wrong way against a fish's scales." However, as he (like everyone else) settled into the lockdowns, he began to feel a great degree of gratitude for his circumstances:

> The resulting seclusion that accompanied the pandemic lockdown and subsequent work-from-home allowances was a positive one for me. My job moved to working from home which was great for the recharge and safety that at-home work can provide. Unexpectedly, it served me well by forcing me to become more self-sufficient in a profession that requires a degree of confidence in one's own expertise. I found that I had really been relying on my boss's knowledge base to cover for safety in situations that should have required my own grit or confidence. I have a great boss who doesn't find it a burden that I would come to him with all sorts of questions. During the pandemic and working from home I found myself needing to fall back on fundamentals to do my job. Being home allowed time for reflective thinking that life in twenty-first century America doesn't typically allow. Pre-pandemic life would be just demanding enough, or many times just distracting enough, that the hard work often accompanying reflective thinking or large-scale conceptual planning wouldn't be worth the effort — at least not in that moment. Feeling rushed, stressed, tired, or distracted would triumph over boredom. The pandemic gave a certain amount of good boredom that things like a 9–5 job or your cell phone have robbed many of. [7]

Brett's expressed gratitude for the greater self-sufficiency it bought him at this job was one comment that I repeatedly heard among those I spoke to. However, it was the second part of Brett's statement about having more time for reflective thinking that surely resonated with many of us during that time. Simply put, without ample time for spirited self-reflection, we cannot evolve into the high spiritual beings that we are all destined to be. For many, what the public health crisis provided was a time to detach from the incessant grind of the 9–5.

In the summer of 2020, I can recall having several uplifting conversations with my good friend Aaron about how grateful he was to finally have paid time off (Aaron was one of the countless millions of people out of work during that time who received expanded unemployment benefits) to reflect on his own personal journey. Prior to that event, Aaron had been a barista at a small coffee bar once owned by my dear and beautiful friends Adam and Tasha. During his time off from work Aaron began exploring his own inner space and as the weeks turned into months, he ultimately decided to leave our friends' café and go back to school to pursue a career in the culinary arts. For my friend then, the most recent pandemic served as a major turning point in his life that, to this day, he remains grateful for.

Looking back now at that difficult point in time, we can find much that we were grateful for. For much of that period, the situation in the nation and throughout the world appeared very bleak. However, that crisis period also provided us with an invaluable opportunity to reflect upon what is truly important in our lives. Personally speaking, I can honestly say that the experience of lockdowns helped me to greater appreciate my good health, my personal relationships, and having the beauty of Mother Nature right out my front door. But most of all, I think it taught me to have far more gratitude for the preciousness of life. I also suspect that many of you feel the same way. From our own personal experiences with death and dying, social isolation, and economic hardship came an even greater gratitude for one very noteworthy thing: the beauty of genuine human connection.

I don't know about you, but since that trying event, I witnessed a certain quality of lightheartedness, much more laughter, and an overflowing expression of love shared between people. To top it all off, I also noticed that a growing number of us appear to have come to the realization that it's the quality of spirit that matters most in our connection with others. Maybe it's just due to the pack of kind hippie souls that I mostly run with, but I have personally experienced more profound instances of human connection in unexpected places following the lockdowns than before. In turn, these experiences have fed the spring of gratitude for life within me. One such extended occurrence took place at the tail end of the most recent pandemic that I think perfectly captures the depths of gratitude for the spirit of human connection that we all share.

The Lodge of Gratitude

Back in late January of 2022, I learned that the college I worked for was forcing my return to Colorado for face-to-face classes. During that time, I had been living in a small but beloved mountain town in North Carolina — twenty-two hours across the country. I fought tooth and nail to prevent my return to face-to-face classes. I made the data-driven case that my student success and satisfaction rates while teaching virtually were exceptional. I also pointed out that the college administration played favorites in deciding which faculty members to whom they granted remote teaching extensions. I even made (what I thought was) a credible argument that forcing my return to campus was retaliation for my obtaining legal aid from a prominent free speech organization in response to that college's censorship of one of my talks. The fact was, that while I loved exploring the majestic Rocky Mountains, I loved the lush and ancient Southern Appalachian Mountains even more. After all, I had forged many beautiful and enduring friendships in that little town, and I was determined to stay. The valuable Buddhist practice of non-attachment could be damned!

Of course, I lost my case to remain teaching online and I returned to Colorado for the spring semester of 2022. As a side note: right now, I know many of you are probably thinking, "Come on Forrest, give me a break. Really? You resisted going back to the Colorado Rockies with its magnificent alpine vistas, legal cannabis, and crisp mountain air? Oh, how hard it must have been for you!"

In any case, on February 1 of that year, I and my long-term partner, Rose, packed up our bags and our two beloved pet-children (Abbie and Luna) and headed west to Colorado. During the first three months there everything was difficult. We couldn't find any stable footing with housing, and we ended up bouncing back and forth between six different apartments. In that same time span, I encountered great hostility on my return to campus because of my unpopular beliefs about what I perceived to be a divisive and disempowering ideology of victimhood promoted on campus by college administrators and faculty. At the end of those three months, I also learned that I was being terminated by the college for openly expressing those same unpopular beliefs. So, I had packed up my entire life and moved halfway across the country for a job that fired me less than three months later. The Universe can certainly have a rascally sense of humor!

During our first ninety days in Colorado, Rose's car accident was by far the hardest thing that happened to us. One day while driving in Boulder, Colorado, a car ran right through a stop sign and crashed into her. In the immediate aftermath of the accident, Rose suffered serious neurological issues. Being unable to work, the financial pressure fell on me. Predictably, this difficult event led to significant stress in our relationship.

Looking back now, my whole reaction to Rose's accident was a reminder that I was still lost in my own worldly attachment to money. In retrospect, it is also amazing to me that after Rose's accident, I allowed my own concerns over finances to overshadow what should have been my own genuine gratitude that she had survived the crash. All in all, our unstable housing situation, me losing my job, and Rose's car accident added up to one hell of a difficult time. But then, like a storm at sea suddenly receding to make way for the patiently waiting sun, a period in my life that I am now so grateful for emerged out of the dark foreboding skies.

For the sixth time in twelve weeks, we were forced to move once more. However, this time our pack of four wound up at a most interesting and healing place. We stayed at a rustic, but mystical lodge nestled in the forests of the Rocky Mountains north of Boulder, Colorado. The thirteen-room lodge sat on the crest of a spectacular mountain at 8,700 feet above sea level and had breathtaking views of the continental divide and the snow-capped peaks of the surrounding Indian Peaks Wilderness. Each morning, walking out of my very humble 300-square-foot abode felt like taking steps into a lost alpine paradise. Having already been relieved of my teaching duties, I spent much of my time at the lodge hiking as much of the vast wilderness in the area as possible. I also happily explored the funky and authentic hippie town of Nederland (near where the lodge was located). To say I fit like a glove in that tiny 1500-person community of "Ned" (as it is affectionally called by locals) is an understatement. Between the 1960s good-vibes feel of the town and the inspiring nature out my front door, I was in heaven. However, it was the genuine connections forged with the people I met at the lodge that cemented my feelings of joy in a soulful foundation of gratitude.

There was Paul, an eccentric but very kind man who had just turned fifty. Paul, who described himself as "the hippie from Alabama," moved into the room directly next to me only days after our own move. Paul, who is a supremely talented artist, was undoubtedly the one person most responsible for transforming the lodge into a real community with his upbeat energy and sense of humor. During his one-month stay, Paul and I engaged in several spontaneous jam sessions together and exchanged our favorite music with one another. In that one month I learned more about folk music (reggae is my true love!) than I ever knew before. Beyond the music though, Paul and I shared profound moments together. We discussed everything from death and dying, to love, to who or what we thought God was. From our many conversations together, I came away feeling that Paul was a tremendously compassionate being who truly cared about the well-being of all people. But like all of us (certainly myself included), Paul wrestled with his own inner demons. His own demon happened to be alcohol. Toward the end of his month stay at the lodge, Paul's drinking spiraled out of control, and he courageously checked himself into a rehab center down the mountain in Boulder. To this day, I keep in regular contact with Paul and keep my fingers crossed that he has remained sober. His kind and generous soul left an indelible mark upon me.

David was another memorable character from the lodge who briefly came into my life. David was a wanderer in the true Jack Kerouac sense and had lived all over the country. Like Paul, David was a very kind, fun, and thoughtful person who deeply contemplated his own life and felt drawn to nature. During the month when our paths crossed, I came to learn that David was going through a profound period of personal suffering. His father had suddenly died the week before we met. For many months he and his wife had also been separated by an ocean as she tried to heal from her own drug addiction in Hawaii where her father lived. Like Paul, David and I shared many impromptu jam sessions and moments of laughter and tears.

Aside from Paul and David, there were several other incredible souls who wandered into that lodge. Each had their own unique stories to tell and rich life experiences to share. Perhaps that was the connecting point between all the wonderfully eclectic people I met at that lodge: rich life experiences. Each of the beings I met had lived mostly non-traditional lives, suffered, and learned through hard knocks like in the case of Shannon, an eccentric music lover filled with wisdom who overcame a five-year stint in prison while he was a young man. During my time at the lodge, I gained an overwhelming sense of gratitude for the very sacredness of human connection. After enduring a frenetic three months on the road spent in relative isolation, finding a community felt incredibly uplifting, fulfilling, and meaningful.

Amid the forming of community at that healing place, something obvious occurred to me: the enforced lockdowns and social distancing that we all collectively experienced starved us of genuine human affection. So, when we all came back together, sincere feelings of gratitude emerged, creating an ocean of appreciation for the power of human connection. Other people I spoke to came to notice this same overflowing gratitude for the sanctity of our relationships. Leila Hancock, an editor/researcher and daughter of the best-selling author Graham Hancock, noted the following in an email exchange with me:

> On a personal level, despite all the suffering that resulted, there seems to be a heightened collective joyfulness that I have experienced at music events and festivals. Also, there is an eagerness to seize the moment, e.g., a massive increase in weddings. I will be going to five this summer![8]

I suspect that many of us experienced this same sense of "collective joyfulness" that Leila expressed.

Finding Gratitude in Our Lives

Beginning during the most recent pandemic I began keeping a gratitude journal. I had never been this specific with journaling before. But I felt the time was right to begin recording one or two things that I felt gratitude for each day. As I started recording my grateful thoughts, as I liked to call them, I noticed that what I felt gratitude for ran the gamut from the mundane to more heavier themes. For example, my first entry in the journal reads:

> Today I am grateful to look out my window and see the mountains greeting me. They (the mountains) bring me so much peace and joy and are a constant reminder of the glorious nature of our Creator.

And on day five of the journal exercise I wrote:

> Today I am grateful for my good health and for the ability to hike through the woods each day. I acknowledge that many people do not have this same ability to do so, and I feel tremendous gratitude that I am able to stroll through the green oasis uninhibited.

And on the sixtieth day of the exercise when I and my partner were without a home and were forced to live out of a hotel for five nights while on the road in Colorado I wrote:

> Today I am grateful for the fact that I have a roof over my head. I am aware that one more difficult turn of events could cast us out into the streets. Then we might really learn what it is truly like to be homeless. Thank God for this hotel.

The idea of starting a gratitude journal may sound cliché to some, but I assure you that it has helped me navigate our post-pandemic world with more understanding and gratitude. Since starting the journal, I also feel like I am learning to take things less for granted, such as good health and access to basic goods like clean water, air, and food. But one of the greatest benefits from starting a gratitude journal is that it pulls us out of our own egoic way of thinking that sees ourselves as victims of circumstance. When we consciously set out to cultivate gratitude in our day-to-day lives, we come to see the ample opportunities for personal growth that emerge out of any trying life experience.

Now, whenever I hear someone complain that they are a victim of this or that circumstance, I listen quietly with my heart wide open to their predicament. But when they finish and ask me my thoughts, I reply with the following questions: "But for what are you grateful? And what are the lessons that you learned through your adversity?" Gratitude profoundly transforms our own relationship with suffering. When we acknowledge feelings of gratitude within us, we come to re-perceive even the worst events in our lives as grist for the mill. Was not all the suffering that we experienced during that time exactly that?

Chapter Three Key Takeaways

- Due to our ego minds, we have the tendency to take the things that really matter in this life for granted like our health, relationships, and our inherent connection to the natural world and each other.

- Gratitude is ground zero for all spiritual work and the foundation of both humility and positivity.

- In various ways, the most recent pandemic helped us foster greater gratitude in our lives.

- The added time we all had during the lockdowns to contemplate our lives and relationship to Spirit is one way that it helped us foster greater gratitude.

- Another source of gratitude that we discovered during that challenging period was the value of our human connections.

- The gratitude that we experienced during and especially in the aftermath of that chaotic time can be incorporated into our spiritual routines through practices like starting a gratitude journal.

- Cultivating gratitude helps us find our reservoir of faith within and helps us transcend personal suffering.

Chapter Three Meditation

Find a comfortable position seated either upright or with legs crossed. Now close your eyes and tune into your breath. Breathe in and breathe out. As you inhale and exhale cross your hands over your heart and picture the moment of a glorious sunrise. As the Sun lights up the gorgeous morning sky, feel its luminous rays illuminate your face and body. Soak up the Sun's healing light and let it fill your whole being with its revitalizing power. The Sun's light is transcendent. The Sun's light is divine. The Sun's light is what sustains you. Give thanks to this light. And then give thanks to the darkness that preceded it. For deep within the recesses of your soul, know that without the darkness, the light you cherish and honor would have no meaning. Continue to breathe in and out. While still holding the image of the Sun's rays in your mind, repeat the following mantra to yourself: "Out of the darkness comes the Sun's light and for this I am grateful." Repeat this mantra again and again: "Out of the darkness comes the Sun's light and for this I am grateful." Give thanks once more to the Sun's light. Give thanks once more to the darkness. Before opening your eyes bow your head three times to the light. Then bow your head three times to the darkness. Open your eyes.

OM.

FOUR
Courage to Chase Your Dreams

The Story of a Hiker and His Search for Greatness

I like to spend as much time as possible hiking in the mountains. The solitude, reflection, fresh air, and communion with nature are my favorite things about being out in the wild. The storied Appalachian Trail crosses within twenty minutes of where I live. Frequently, while hiking on the "AT," as it's known by Appalachian Trail hikers, I will encounter a "thru-hiker" (one attempting to hike the entire 2,181 trail end to end). I have found that taking the time to talk to these folks is always worth the brief intrusion into my own solo experience in nature. These individuals are filled with so much passion, dedication, and spirit that conversing with them never fails to uplift my own day.

Sometime during the lockdowns, I crossed paths with a thru-hiker on a local summit. As we introduced ourselves to one another he told me his name was "Noble." Noble was his given trail name (it is a time-honored tradition in the Appalachian Trail community that every thru-hiker is given a trail name by another thru-hiker), and he went by that rather than his real moniker. He excitedly explained that this was his first attempt at hiking the AT but that he had successfully completed the other two major long-distance trails in the United States — the 2,650-mile Pacific Crest Trail (PCT) and the 3,100-mile Continental Divide Trail (CDT).

For Noble, completing the AT would earn him the very rare (only 440 hikers since 1994 have achieved the feat) and remarkably difficult honor of the "Triple Crown." A Triple Crown is when a hiker completes each of the three major long-distance trails in the United States. Each of the efforts must be documented and the few who complete the monumental challenge are awarded with plaques of distinction each fall at a banquet organized by the Appalachian Long-Distance Hikers Association (ALDHA).

During our brief interaction, I remember asking Noble (who was fifty-five years old at the time and gave off the vibe of having found total inner peace) why he desired to attempt this inspiring feat amid a major pandemic that kept roughly ninety percent of the hikers who annually embark on the trek off the trail. A huge smile broke out across his face as he simply replied, "Because it's my destiny and I am the shaper of it."

After a few minutes, I wished him good luck on his incredible journey north to his destination of Mount Katahdin in Maine. We then went our separate ways. All I could think about on my way back down the mountain to my car was his inspiring words: "Because it's my destiny and I am the shaper of it."

I thought to myself how Noble embodied the very essence of courage. His quest reminds me a lot of Paulo Coelho's mystical character, Santiago, in the best-selling book *The Alchemist*. In that celebrated novel, Santiago goes on a long and epic pilgrimage in search of a hidden treasure only to discover that the journey itself was his real destiny. Noble's words and example should serve as inspiration that even during extreme periods of fear and anxiety (such as during a pandemic) we can still find the courage to chase our dreams.

Dreams Worth Chasing

At the height of the government shutdowns, John, a friend of mine from Colorado, shared his dreams with me while on a gorgeous hike through the mountains together. In the year leading up to the viral outbreak, this incredibly talented sound engineer and music booker spent around eighty hours a week working at a music venue. While he found his work satisfying, he confided in me that the long hours and breakneck pace of booking bands six nights a week and running sound for those same acts had taken an emotional toll on him.

Like many skilled workers in the entertainment industry, John suddenly found himself unemployed when all bars and music venues were forced to shut down. But he was one of the lucky ones. In contrast to the countless millions of desperate laid-off workers that would follow, John experienced a smooth transition to the unemployment rolls. He related to me that the time away from his job provided him with a greater sense of balance and fulfillment in his own life. It has also strengthened his relationship with his wife. Most of all, John's hiatus away from the daily grind gave him the courage to chase his dreams and live his life to the fullest. Eventually, John and his wife followed their dream to live in an RV and moved off to a remote and beautiful track of land outside of Moab, Utah.

In the aftermath of that period, stories like John's have increasingly grown in number. It appears that many people came to the realization that life is short and that they had better use their time wisely chasing their dreams. Having stared our fear of death in the face, our collective experience has carved out an existential cross-roads that we have all been called on to navigate. Despite the immense emotional and physical damage left in its wake, the public health crisis proved to be something of a blessing for many people who felt trapped in the societal machine for far too long. The conditions were ripe to pour our time and energy into pursuits that more meaningfully serve the higher qualities of the human spirit.

For those people like Dylan F., a former touring musician turned mushroom farmer, the period of lockdowns led him to reassess his life and find the courage to deepen his relationship with nature and follow his dream to start his own farm. In Dylan's own inspiring words:

> The timing of the pandemic just happened to coincide with an already dynamic transition in life. After spending almost ten years as a touring guitar player for a rock band, I was forced to reassess and adapt to the end of an era. We played the last show as The Delta Saints in the fall of 2018.
>
> It was then I decided to return to college and pursue a degree in biology. I chose a rigorous class schedule, and by the start of the pandemic I was just over a semester away from graduating.
>
> At the start of the pandemic, there was the obvious fear and confusion that persisted everywhere; however, I was able to continue my college courses online and through Zoom™, as well as continued doing research at the university under an NSF grant.
>
> I chose to get a second job at a local organic farm that summer of 2020 (while continuing the research grant on my days off from the farm). It was through this difficult and rewarding venture that I fell in love with agriculture and food production and decided to start my own business cultivating gourmet and medicinal mushrooms. I was able to practice full-scale mushroom production and revitalize the current mushroom program at the farm. My partner, Mickenzie, and I were also refining our personal home farming techniques at our urban farmstead (home). We created a quarter acre of bountiful organic vegetable production in the backyard of our neighborhood home in Nashville. [9]

Dylan F. continued:

> We had so many new experiments and projects during the hardest points of the lockdowns that we hardly noticed what was going on. We were able to stay isolated or outside almost the entire time, and that kept the cabin fever or conflict at bay.
>
> By the beginning of the spring in 2021, I graduated from college majoring in biology and minoring in chemistry; we officially launched our new mushroom company, Nashville Farmacy; we bought property in the country to start our permanent farmstead; and I got engaged to my amazing partner. I know the pandemic has been so hard for so many, but our staying busy and finding courage to work toward our life goals made the best of the situation. The discomforts and changes forced upon us through isolation, confusion, and lifestyle shifts came with the blessing of realization. It made us focus only on the most important things and look inward at what we truly wanted out of life. We wanted a loving connection with our friends and family, security, access to good health and nutrition, environments that cultivate joy and creativity, and land that would help deepen our connection to nature. We have found all of these things through our recent efforts, and the pandemic played no small role. [10]

The Three Mindsets

In response to the most recent pandemic, there emerged three distinct mindsets among people. The first were those who responded to the health-related impacts of the crisis with extreme fear and anxiety. Throughout that time, individuals who assumed this mindset were more prone to consuming the overwhelmingly fearful health narratives peddled by predominantly left-of-center media outlets, meticulously followed health safety protocols (even in those cases when they conflicted with the latest scientific data like in the case of the efficacy of vaccines), and were generally paralyzed by an agonizing fear of death. For this group of people, the contagion presented such a direct threat that life as they knew it came to a screeching halt. In other words, many people simply stopped living and instead clung to what was safe and familiar. While such a mindset undoubtedly contributed to our country's declining mental health in the U.S., the extreme fear and anxiety that these individuals felt is perfectly understandable and relatable. After all, if you were over sixty years old or suffered with a debilitating ailment like diabetes or cancer, that was a particularly terrifying time. And if you experienced the loss of a close friend or relative or nearly died yourself from the virus, your fear was only heightened.

Yet, a second mindset emerged in response to the viral contagion. This one reflected a belief that the virus itself was largely overblown by power-hungry politicians and profit-driven media companies seeking to use the public health crisis to further their own control over the people. To a very large extent, all of this was true. A compelling case could be made that that event led to the dangerous overreach of government power and control over the people (for example, the undeniably authoritarian vaccine mandates, government shutdowns of private businesses, and enforced closure of houses of worship). However, in the end, people with this mindset also lived riddled with fear. Whereas the first mindset genuinely reflected fear of the health-related consequences of the virus, the second reflected fear of the political-related consequences of the pandemic. While people with this politically driven emphasis showed little fear of dying from the illness or passing it to others, they still lived in fear. So much fear in fact, that numerous individuals ascribed to absurd and over-the-top conspiracy theories about the validity of the existence of the virus itself. Of course, such fear and paranoia about the political impacts of the pandemic were also peddled by media outlets — in this case, those that were right-of-center.

Gratefully, a third mindset emerged that totally transcended the worldly theatre of fear and paranoia and instead approached it from a perspective of spiritual growth and personal empowerment. People who ascribed to this mindset were all over the spectrum regarding their own levels of concern about the health and political impacts of the virus. However, what they shared was a desire to use this once-in-a-lifetime event to evolve in their consciousness. The following are some common questions that people with this personal growth mindset asked during the most recent pandemic:

- In what ways will living through this event help me become a more compassionate and wiser being?
- How can I use this period to better transcend my own fear of death and live more presently in the moment?
- What spiritual practices (such as prayer or meditation) can I pursue during this time that will bring me closer to God, the One?
- How has my experience during this time redefined my personal hopes, dreams, and aspirations?
- In these times, how can I best be of service to humanity and Earth?

While writing this book, I talked with countless people who met the challenges posed by the pandemic through diligently working on themselves. For Nick P., a brilliant musician from the Great Smoky Mountains of North Carolina, that event helped him overcome his long-running drug addiction and develop a deep and lasting personal relationship with God. Through several moving conversations, Nick shared how the stresses of life during a pandemic only increased his own suffering and led him back down into a dark hole of substance abuse. However, unlike his past attempts at getting sober, he finally succeeded thanks in no small part to the intervention and loving support extended to him by family and friends. In his own words, Nick related how grateful he is for the life-altering time that he spent in a Christ-centered rehabilitation center:

> My time in rehab gave me a chance to re-examine the roots of my pain and those destructive habits that fed my addiction. Most importantly, rehab gave me the opportunity to get right with God again and make him the focal point of my own life. [11]

Since exiting rehab, Nick has completely transformed his life. While he had long been a "functioning addict" in the sense that he had held down a respected and well-paying job as an electrician, he made the choice to double down on his lifelong pursuit of music. He also dropped all the negative friends in his life who fed his addiction and began to surround himself with more positive and uplifting influences. In addition, Nick began to regularly attend church, committed himself to an intense daily fitness regimen, and relocated to have a fresh start. Still sober, Nick's inspiring story is a testament to the power of finding personal courage during an otherwise difficult time.

For Elijah Dicks, an accomplished professor and former colleague of mine, the period of lockdowns provided a unique opportunity to further grow his courage (Elijah definitely has deep reserves of courage in his bones as evidenced by one remarkable occurrence when he heroically risked his own life to save an elderly man from a car when that victim drove off the edge of a mountain and crashed onto the banks of a river) and start a YouTube™ channel centered on personal growth and healthy male empowerment. Through dedicated time and effort, Elijah managed to skillfully produce a successful and uplifting channel that has garnered millions of views. Elijah, who has always extolled and lived the values of courage, faith, and individual accountability, noted that the most recent pandemic gave humanity a large dose of adversity with which to work. And that adversity, according to him, is not something that we should ever shy away from meeting:

> I have always said, you shouldn't wish for a trouble-free life. Rather, you should pray for the strength to overcome the adversity that we will all inevitably face. Only through adversity can you be manifested into the strongest iteration of yourself. [12]

I personally align with and see great value in Elijah's comments. Unfortunately, the most recent pandemic revealed a sharp disconnect between those who chose to respond to that event by embracing adversity while others did not. At the height of the contagion, when all classes at the college were being taught virtually, I delivered a virtual campus-wide talk about how we could mindfully use the circumstances of that event for our own personal growth. Around seventy people attended the talk and boy, let me tell you, my emphasis on self-empowerment was not well received at all! The basic premise of that lecture was that we, as conscious actors, have the power to choose how we decide to respond to that adversity-filled time. I argued that we were being conditioned by societal authorities (such as the government and media) to react to the crisis with extreme fear and paranoia.

While I was especially careful to emphasize the very real suffering that people had endured, I asked my audience the following question: "In the face of such profound suffering, how do we choose to respond?" My argument then, as it still is now, was that moments of extreme adversity make us stronger. In that talk, I explained that the pandemic could help us foster more gratitude in our day-to-day lives, make peace with the inevitability of death, and even deepen our wisdom. In short, I incorporated some of the very lessons from this book into that presentation.

A few people in the audience enthusiastically accepted my invitation to adopt a courageous personal growth mindset during that time. However, most people in attendance reacted quite negatively to my suggestion to let go, let God, and embrace the highest versions of ourselves. One very vocal academic psychologist accused me of peddling a "male White privileged" perspective and said that a mindset of personal and spiritual growth was simply not feasible for marginalized groups in America to adopt. Another academic critic, in this case a self-described "radical feminist," said my self-growth perspective was evidence of "toxic positivity." I almost toppled over when I heard that one! And yet another naysayer accused my personal growth perspective as being out of touch with "oppressed colonized peoples" in America. To say the least, the ideas I expressed that day were met with a very icy reception.

What I discovered through this experience was that fear has a deeply disempowering impact on our ability to respond to adversity. While speaking to that group of mostly self-identified "social justice warriors," the only emotions I felt emanating from the audience were those of extreme fear and misplaced anger. Admittedly, my initial reaction to their open hostility was one of judgment. I thought to myself about how sad it was that they gave into so much fear and squandered a valuable opportunity to discover the courage to look within themselves. Today, I can see how misplaced my own judgment was. Now all I feel when I think back on that day is genuine compassion for the rough seas that they, just like I, are attempting to navigate in the best way they know how.

Changing Perspectives

An interesting phenomenon emerged in the wake of the most recent pandemic. Young workers everywhere (at least in the Western world) quit their jobs en masse. In fact, so many people resigned from their jobs all at once that at the time the media dramatically dubbed this event "the Great Resignation." However, behind this liberating movement there was an implicit understanding that the talking heads failed to capture. This understanding was that the culture's promises of fulfillment through the accumulation of money and endless consumption just wasn't cutting it. For a short period, it seemed that millions of young people began to see through the societal illusion that we are all programmed from childhood on to accept. You know that illusion as well as I: go into debt to obtain a corporatized education to make money for someone else, buy a house and some nice things, drive a flashy car (or two) and THEN finally start to live life just as your body begins its decline in old age.

Many people I spoke to were eager to share their own personal stories of quitting their jobs to pursue one dream or another. Engineers, teachers, restaurant staff, and office assistants. The list goes on. The one thing that was most apparent through all my communications with these workers was a realization that life is too short and precious to be wasted on the pursuit of material gain at the expense of living. Perhaps that is why so many people I spoke to opted out of the many trappings of homeownership and instead bought and outfitted vans to see more of the country. It also explains why so many of these same people expressed a genuine desire to live more simply and delve into the spiritual side of life. For those like Cassandra S., an engineer from Tampa, Florida, the period of lockdowns sparked these desires:

> When my job went virtual, I suddenly had more time to dive deeper into myself...my own being. And what I saw was that the way I had been living up to that point wasn't conducive to real happiness for me. So, with the ten hours or so per week that I now had back from my commute to and back from work, I found a yoga center and began that practice. And after four blissful months of twice-weekly yoga sessions, I made the decision to sell my house and give van life a try. At the same time, I also decided to enroll in yoga teacher training and pursue a new life goal to become a yoga instructor. Without the circumstances of that event (the pandemic), I am not sure if I would have ever found the courage to quit my well-paying job and sell my house. [13]

I can personally relate to Cassandra's story. During the period of lockdowns, I began to seriously question once again what my own life purpose was. To me, it was plain to see that teaching in academia was no longer in harmony with my own journey. The greater time spent in solitude and reflection gave me the clarity to see that working in the colleges was creating more frustration than happiness and that I had to make a change. Simply going through the mechanical motions of teaching someone else's curriculum every semester no longer brought the same degree of fulfillment that I had experienced earlier in my "career."

During that time, I turned ever deeper into three great loves of mine: writing, making music, and spending time in nature. The added space for inner contemplation that I experienced, showed me that my personal destiny was to be a spiritual teacher and that writing, music, and nature were to be the channels that I teach through. Far from giving up teaching, I realized that all that was happening was that I was liberating myself from the constraints of institutionalized education so that I could freely practice my craft for the first time. Without that period of societal upheaval, I am not sure if I would have had the courage to evolve as a teacher and follow my higher calling. It is important to remember that each of us has a higher calling. And each of us are fully capable of realizing it. All we must do is find the courage within us to chase our dreams.

Chapter Four Key Takeaways

- The recent pandemic provided an important opportunity for people to reflect on their own lives and question if they were living in accord with their own inner truth.

- The time spent at home away from their jobs helped shift people's focus from material to spiritual pursuits.

- One result of this seismic shift in life perspective was that many people grew the courage to chase their personal dreams.

- The specifics of these dreams differed from person to person. For some, living off the land or embracing "van life" represented a return to simplicity. Yet for others, chasing their dreams meant quitting their jobs and re-devoting their time to spiritual practice and the attainment of self-realization.

- Unfortunately, during that time, many people opted not to chase their dreams due to extreme fear.

- This extreme fear surfaced in two ways among people: through the constant worry of getting sick and through paranoia about the motives of political leaders in charge during that public health crisis. On the surface, those who lived in fear of getting sick from the virus and those who lived in fear of political power appeared to conflict with one another. However, both groups ironically shared the same emphasis in projecting fear.

- The way to overcome such extreme fear is through tapping into the reservoir of boundless courage that lies within. Only then can we begin to pursue our higher purpose in life.

Chapter Four Meditation

Find a comfortable position seated either upright or with legs crossed. Now close your eyes and tune into your breath. Breathe in and breathe out. As you inhale and exhale imagine a purple antenna attached to the top of your head. Then imagine that antenna gradually extending up toward the sky from your crown chakra, through Earth's atmosphere, and into outer space. This purple antenna is your light of courage. It is your transmitter of dream manifestation. Now, as you continue to focus on your breath, bring all your life's dreams to mind. Don't hold back. Whatever dreams and aspirations you have for this incarnation, hold them in your mind. Send these thought forms of your dreams straight from your mind through the purple antenna and into the celestial heavens above. As you release your dreams into the timeless void of space repeat the following prayer to yourself: "By the grace of the Divine Universe, may my dreams be realized." Repeat this prayer over and over: "By the grace of the Divine Universe, may my dreams be realized." And so shall it be. While continuing to repeat the prayer, slowly imagine the purple antenna retracting back through the galaxies, planets, and stars, then through Earth's atmosphere, until it merges once again with your crown chakra. You are the dreams that you manifest into reality.

OM.

FIVE
Surviving by Faith

A Personal Story of Faith

MANY years back, my partner Rose and I went through a difficult ordeal. Shortly after moving from the city to the mountains, we suddenly found ourselves forced to move out of our first mountain rental. For three and a half months, the two of us had wandered the beautiful trails that surrounded the cabin where we lived, paid homage to a glorious waterfall that was right outside our back door, and frequented cows that grazed in the adjacent pastures. Never had either of us felt so connected to nature. However, soon after moving into the cabin, Rose grew severely ill. We soon discovered that there was a massive black mold build-up in the foundation of the house. We had no other choice but to abandon the dwelling and head back to the city of Nashville, Tennessee where we had been living for years prior.

The move back home was heartbreaking for the two of us. We cried and mourned the loss of our beloved mountains. To make matters worse, our landlords at that time refused to take responsibility for Rose's illness when we tried to recoup money for her medical costs. In the weeks following our sudden departure from the cabin, we twice made the 5–hour drive back and forth from Nashville in the span of a half month. Our hope was to find a new rental. On our first trip back to Western North Carolina, we were primarily consumed with moving our belongings out of the cottage. During this four-day period, we stayed with a friendly young couple who we met through an Airbnb™ website. On the second day, they learned of our desire to remain in the mountains and offered to rent their house out to us. We were beyond ecstatic! *What luck*, we thought. However, it was never meant to be. Only two days after our return to Nashville, we received an email from the couple saying that they couldn't rent to us after all. We were totally bummed. Two weeks later, we traveled once more to the mountains to check out two rentals that we had found on online. But neither came as advertised. That night we headed back to our hotel room and lamented our circumstances.

The next morning, Rose and I had a conversation in the hotel room about all the recent adversity we had endured. We spoke of her ongoing illness due to the mold, our having to leave the mountains, and the long-term prospects of returning to the city. As we stood around in the hotel room and discussed our predicament, Rose mentioned in passing how most hotels in the United States place Bibles in the drawers of hotel rooms. She motioned for me to check the drawer. As if on cue, I picked up the Holy Bible that was in our own drawer and I flipped it open to a random page. The section it turned to be was the first page of the Book of Job. We looked at each other in awe. If we needed proof from the horse's mouth that our suffering wasn't for naught, there it was.

As "disciples of the Universe" (a wonderful phrase coined by my wise friend Ed), we both got the message loud and clear! IT seemed to be conveying the very point of the legendary parable: suffering tests your faith in God and those who keep their faith in the Divine will always be blessed and cared for. Adding to the surreal feeling of this moment was that in the three weeks leading up to this event we had been finding great solace in the lyrics of a song written by our good friend. The song was titled, "Cry to Jah" and was about the biblical Job and his dramatic encounters with suffering. *Incredible!* we thought.

A few days later, when we recounted this synchronicity to our dear friends Jonny and Lynn from the mountains, Jonny summed it up perfectly in saying, "It sounds like God spoke directly to you through those pages."

The Power of Faith

Faith is a beautiful thing. It can be compared to a budding flower, intuitively growing into its purpose to inspire and give life. Faith is the bedrock of hope. For without it, our moments of suffering would appear to be without meaning. On the spiritual path, we could probably all agree that compassion, positivity, humility, and a sincere desire to liberate oneself from the illusion of separateness are each key qualities that any seeker on the path must cultivate within before coming to God. However, as a demonstration of its power, it is faith alone that sustains each of these qualities. For example, true compassion can only be said to arise when you arrive at the place within you — and I arrive at the place within me — that just intuitively knows that we are all connected in Spirit as one. Once you and I both know this (and I mean when we really feel it within our souls), how can we not have compassion for each other? After all, if we are all one, then that means that we are all soul brothers and sisters.

Like compassion, faith also sustains the light of positivity. For what is positivity but a faithful mindset that life has both a deeper meaning and a higher purpose? Faith, too, sustains our capacity to respond to moments of personal suffering with greater humility through guiding us to surrender to a power beyond ourselves. Finally, without the faith to sustain us, the numerous pitfalls on the spiritual path that we all encounter would simply be too much for us all to bear and we would give up at once our desire for liberation. But during life's difficult moments when we find ourselves in the dark night of the soul, faith lights our path forward and helps us see that those very pitfalls we endure play a crucial role in our journey of awakening.

There is a remarkable story about the power of faith that Ram Dass relates to us in the pages of his beautiful book, *Paths to God: Living the Bhagavad Gita*. This story was told to him by the great Indian holy man Swami Muktananda:

> Krishna, at one stage of his incarnation as an avatar, was a beautiful young boy (something you'll need to know to understand this tale). Now there was a great student of the Bhagavad Gita (arguably the greatest of all the Hindu holy books that centers on the highest spiritual teachings of Krishna as God incarnate), an old man. He was so intent on studying the Gita that he had stopped doing all of his work; he wouldn't do anything but read the Gita all day long. Soon he and his wife were without food. His wife was understandably very harsh with him saying, "You have a duty to go out and bring food home for the family." She kept pressing him, making his life very difficult, but he'd just go off into the woods and study the Gita every day. One day, as he sat in the woods studying the Gita, the old man came across a line in the book in which Krishna said, "If you offer all of your devotion to me, you need worry about nothing in the world. It will all be taken care of." And the old man thought, *Well, isn't that a peculiar line? I mean, here I am, totally devoted to the Gita, to Krishna, but my wife and I have not food, and she's all upset with me. It says right here that if I am devoted to the Gita, everything will be taken care of. Why isn't everything being taken care of? Could there possibly be something wrong with the Gita?* At that point he took out his pen and drew a line through the sentence, because he wasn't sure about it. Now at that exact moment, back at his (the old man's) house, there was a knock at the door. The wife went to the door and there stood a handsome

young man, with bags of rice and of lentils and of flour — huge bags, a supply to last for many months. The wife said, "Who are you? What is all this?" The young man said, "This is for the family of somebody who studies the Gita." As the young man started to carry the bags of food into the house, the wife noticed that his shirt was torn open, and that there was a wound on his chest, with blood oozing out of the wound. She said to him, "What happened? Who did this to you?" He said, "This was done to me by a man studying the Gita out in the woods." He said no more, put down the bags of food, and left. When the husband came back home and saw all the food, he asked his wife about it. She said, "You know, the most peculiar thing happened." She proceeded to tell him about the young man's visit, and she said, "When I looked at him, I saw there was blood coming out of a wound on his chest. And when I asked him how it happened, he said it had been done by a man studying the Gita out in the woods." The old man realized what had happened, and he fainted. Because he saw that when he had underlined the sentence of the book out of his sense of doubt, he had wounded the body of Krishna. [14]

There is so much to unpack from this story as it relates to the power of faith. The purity of the old man's devotion to Krishna summoned what we here in the West would call a "miracle" through the sudden deliverance of life sustaining food by Krishna disguised as the young man. But while the story profoundly captures the transcendent power of cultivating faith in God, it is also something of a cautionary tale for what happens when our faith flickers and doubt creeps in for just a moment. The bodily harm that the old man inflicted on Krishna through his momentary loss of faith symbolizes the harm that we cause to ourselves when we allow our thinking minds to circumvent what we know to be the truth within.

Faith vs. Belief

During the most recent pandemic, countless people began questioning the direction of their own daily routines. Like the 1960s and 70s, one consequence of such widespread questioning was that great skepticism emerged (particularly among those forty years old and younger) about the foundational values of our culture and society. In so many ways, the very context of that time dramatically exposed the sheer hollowness of our institutions, structures, and traditions. The destructive and exploitive tendencies of an economic system focused solely on profit and not real human needs was laid bare for all to see through the egregious profiteering by unaccountable multinational corporations during that crisis. And all the open corruption and mass deception carried out by our political leaders (from both parties) in response to that once-in-a-lifetime event led many to question the legitimacy of our democracy. Of course, the mainstream media's propagandistic coverage (on both sides) of the major social upheavals and events of that time only wound up provoking greater feelings of skepticism and resentment from an already fearful population.

Normally, such widespread questioning of institutional authority is a positive thing because it commonly leads to movements of higher consciousness. However, when movements of higher consciousness just start out, the inner faith of individual seekers within those movements can flicker. When inner faith flickers, people become more susceptible to adopting extremist beliefs of one kind or another. The reason for this is simple: absent an unconditional faith in God or the One, we tend to revert to our programmed response of looking outside rather than within for reassurance. The result is that our intrinsic need for divine connection is replaced by an overidentification with worldly causes and leaders. And as we all surely know by now — it is remarkably easy to be swept away by the fervor of worldly passions.

During the public health crisis, our attachments to extreme belief came to replace genuine faith. Predictably, political demagogues of all stripes were more than willing to exploit the flickering faith of all those who sincerely yearned for a conscious revolution of the spirit. In the end, these demagogues did what demagogues are programmed to do. And that programming is designed to divert our innate drive for divine connection toward divisive political movements like phony social justice activism or overly aggressive nationalism. During that public health crisis, plenty of otherwise good-intentioned people vaulted to the extreme camps of the nation's two major political parties. And the result was more division, conflict, violence, and lack of tolerance for differing viewpoints and perspectives. Those who identified with each of the two extreme ideologies resorted to blaming the other side for exasperating a dramatic event that should have unified all of us beyond the illusion of separateness.

On this point of adopting extreme beliefs, I can recall a highly relatable story that fortunately has a happy ending. The story centers around an inspiring individual I know named Dave C. Dave, who is a brilliant artist that builds art installations for music and art festivals, arrived at an existential crossroads at the start of the most recent pandemic. As fate would have it, Dave found himself in Portland, Oregon only days after a highly charged racial event that rocked both the country and the world. While there, he took on a lover who introduced him to the world of social activism. Before he knew it, Dave was participating in violent nightly street clashes with heavily militarized local police and federal agents. He also began co-mingling with political extremists and even adopted the black bloc attire of the other left-wing street activists that he met. He also began adopting the divisive mindset of those around him by openly denouncing all those on the extreme right of the political spectrum who engaged in sometimes violent counter protests as White supremacists and Brownshirts.

Dave related to me how at first the social movement for racial justice energized him at a point in his life where he felt he lacked direction. However, after spending a night in jail for refusing to disburse during a declared riot by police, Dave began to question his involvement in the movement. He saw how impressionable he could be and how easily it was for his thoughts and behaviors to be manipulated. He also shared with me how easy it is for our thoughts to be molded and manipulated by ideals that are not necessarily our own through the dissemination of information that is intended to manipulate. Now on to the happy ending that I promised! After three months, Dave left Portland and his brief incursion into the world of political radicalism to focus on his own personal and spiritual growth. In retrospect, while his intentions during that time were pure (he was motivated to end racial injustice) he learned the paramount importance of not being seduced by extreme belief, following his own convictions, and most important of all — finding his own inner faith. Today, Dave remains one of the most soulful and reflective people that I have ever met.

Surely, each of us must accept some of the blame for allowing ourselves to be seduced by extreme beliefs that imagines a world of "us" and "them." However, it's not all our fault for why so many of us fell prey to such beliefs during that challenging time. Some of that blame rests on the shoulders of our own religious leaders. The highest purpose of religion should be to inspire us to cultivate genuine faith within ourselves. But to do so, the leaders of our religious traditions must lead by example through displaying the characteristics of genuine love, compassion, and selflessness. This role for our religious leaders is especially important during moments of crisis when collective confusion, fear, and uncertainty frustrate attempts at finding inner faith.

During the viral outbreak, can we honestly say that overall, our religious leaders rose to the occasion to counter all the extremist beliefs at that time? The shocking scandals of corruption and sexual violence that continued to rock official churchdom combined with the precipitous decline in church membership among the youth suggests that the answer to that question is no. If people turn to religion for spiritual comfort and all they find is hypocrisy among the very shepherds who are supposed to inspire them to see that the kingdom of God is truly within them, then they will turn to worldly leaders to fulfill their needs for strength and assurance.

Moving forward, it would be wise if we remembered that faith and belief are not the same thing. Belief says: "Through my rational mind I *think* all is one." Faith says: "Within my soul I *know* all is one." Belief thinks. Faith knows. Belief is fleeting and can easily be broken at the first sign of struggle. The reason why belief is so fragile is because it is a projection of our egos. One of the defining characteristics of the ego is that it views the world through the lens of separation. And, because it sees itself as separate from the one reality, its thoughts are not truly rooted in anything but its own narrow framework of how it "thinks" the world should be. This lack of intuitive knowing explains why belief often produces the extreme perspectives we witnessed. In the absence of a more intuitive and non-dual understanding, we substitute our lack of faith with belief and set out to convert others to validate that false truth for us.

In contrast to belief is faith. Faith is our own conquering of fear through inner surrender. It is born through an intuitive knowing that is strengthened through heartfelt prayer and meditation. Faith finds its expression through all authentic acts of kindness and is also firmly rooted in our own direct experience. Another aspect of faith is that it conveys an eternal quality of truth that does not need to be spoken to convert believers. With faith, one has no desire to proselytize because what is known can only be accessed within. The desire to inspire others through sharing wisdom and baring our souls is a hallmark of faith. The desire to control another's thoughts is a hallmark of belief. Faith is the source of inspiration for the sincerest artists, counselors, and seekers. The latter is too often the motivation for politicians and religious leaders. Faith heals and unites. Belief injures and divides.

Sweet Surrender

One Sunday morning at the tail end of the contagion, I found myself at a beautiful spiritual center in Franklin, North Carolina. The center's membership is an eclectic community of seekers who celebrate their love of Spirit through a blend of Eastern and Western mystical traditions. The guest speaker that day was an inspiring man named Bill. Gratefully, I have gotten to know Bill well over the years through his former role as lead facilitator of the center. As far as I am concerned, Bill is a fully realized being. Though he wouldn't ever say so, his vast range of life experiences (which included ten years of service as a priest on a Native American Reservation in Colorado, a period of heavy alcohol abuse which he overcame, several years spent as a drug and alcohol counselor, as well as two years spent hitchhiking across the nation) made this infinitely wise man the perfect instrument to deliver a message about inner faith and surrender. In that talk delivered before a room full of seekers, Bill acknowledged the uncertain and trying times we were living in and then he proceeded to talk about the importance of surrender. After describing the peaks and valleys of his own spiritual journey, he explained how important but difficult it is to surrender to God and allow IT to work through you as an instrument of divine will. In moving fashion, Bill explained when that moment of inner surrender finally happened for him. In his own words:

> While living on the Reservation I was attempting to turn the mission into a parish. But things on the Reservation were so riddled with addiction that, like all the priests before me, I too fell into addiction. I knew I needed to go to treatment and leave the priesthood. There was so much dysfunction on the Reservation that people living there literally had no place to sleep and in my drunken state I would forget to close the doors to the church, and I would awake in the morning and there would be bodies everywhere sleeping on the floor. There is one moment that stands out to me. I remember lying down (drunk) on the ground wearing nothing but a T-shirt in the middle of the night in November (in Colorado). I was utterly numb to the world, and I suddenly became aware that I was spiritually barren inside. I couldn't pray; nothing would rise up. And in that utter deadness within, these words just came out as if God himself were praying through me: "God, do whatever you want to do with me to make me into the person you most want me to become." I finally felt peace I hadn't felt in a long time. And that prayer became part of my daily life after that. [15]

The powerful moment of surrender that Bill described in that talk is one that probably resonates with many people's experiences during the most recent pandemic. Chris G., a middle school teacher from Salt Lake City, Utah who I spoke to, explained that the circumstances of that event forced him in his own words to "surrender to a higher power." He elaborated:

> At the start of the pandemic, my wife and I heard all the reports on the news about this deadly new virus and I must admit we were completely overwhelmed by fear. For the first two months of lockdown, we, like most people, took every precaution that we could to be safe. We wore masks, limited our exposure in public, kept our distance from others, and even wiped down all our groceries. But following one especially fearful grocery shop when an unmasked man began coughing right in front of me in the checkout line, I suddenly had this realization while sitting down for dinner: I couldn't control anything that was happening. If it was my time to die, it was my time to die. In that moment I then realized that I had to place my faith in a higher power because only he knew how that event would unfold. [16]

Like Bill, Chris G. recalls feeling a wave of peace wash over him upon realizing that his and everyone's fate was really in the hands of God. Again, in his own words:

All I could do was surrender to the moment and trust in my higher power. I can't describe how much peace I felt in surrendering to that which is so much greater than me. From that point on, I still took reasonable precautions to protect myself from the virus, but I no longer lived with excessive fear. I now fully understand the meaning of the biblical phrase, "Faith can move mountains."[17]

Indeed, faith can move mountains. And may we never forget it!

Chapter Five Key Takeaways

- Suffering tests our personal faith.
- Faith alone sustains compassion, positivity, humility, and the desire to liberate oneself from the illusion of separateness.
- True faith summons miracles in our day-to-day lives.
- The most recent pandemic dramatically revealed the flaws in our culture, which in turn spawned a movement of higher consciousness.
- Flickering faith was an emergent feature within this movement of higher consciousness.
- One consequence of our flickering faith was that many otherwise well-intentioned people adopted extreme beliefs.
- The adoption of extreme beliefs especially manifested itself in our politics.
- Our embracing of extreme beliefs results in division, conflict, violence, and a lack of tolerance for opinions that differ from our own.
- The lack of moral leadership by our religious leaders was partly to blame for the emergence of extreme belief during that public health crisis.
- It is important to remember that faith heals and unites, while belief injures and divides.
- Surrendering to a higher power is the path to finding inner peace.
- Faith can move mountains!

Chapter Five Meditation

Find a comfortable position seated either upright or with legs crossed. Now close your eyes and tune into your breath. Breathe in and breathe out. As you inhale and exhale try and recall a being who inspires feelings of divine love like compassion, humility, and wisdom. This being could be alive or disembodied. Now imagine yourself sitting on the ground in the lotus position staring into the eyes of that being seated only a couple feet in front of you. Feel the infinite warmth and unconditional love flowing from that being to you, a seeker of truth and higher knowing. As you bathe in their radiant warmth, realize that there is nothing to be ashamed of and nothing to fear as this being already knows everything about your past, present, and future. For he or she is your inner guru beyond space and beyond time.

Now allow yourself the freedom to surrender your heart to the care of the divine being before you. As you surrender, picture releasing all your anxieties, fears, and worries and repeat the following mantra: "I am the flute by which the breath of God flows through. So may you breathe through me as an expression of your will." Repeat this mantra in your mind repeatedly until its timeless words move from your mind to your lips and finally down to your spiritual heart. Now bow three times to the divine being seated before you and take a moment to acknowledge the sheer miracle of consciousness that brought you and them together in the same sacred space. The moment of your surrender is here. Now open your eyes and be the light that helps all others see that God's kingdom is found within yourself through realizing a faith as boundless as the ocean.

OM.

SIX
Healing through Prayer

Unlocking the Gates of Heaven

THERE **are two** primary channels through which we can unlock the gates of heaven within ourselves. The first is through the power of prayer and the second is through the practice of meditation. Prayer can be thought of as an invocation or act of communion during which we share our faithful intentions and conscious desires with God, the Universe. Meditation is the act of stilling your mind and tuning your soul toward the wisdom of God, the Universe. In the depths of meditation, we learn how to listen for divine guidance within. In accessing this inner space, it is important to understand that prayer and meditation are not dueling counterparts. Just as joy and suffering are part of the same cosmic cycle, so it is between prayer and meditation.

No seeker of truth may be said to truly know the one without the other. Our faithful intentions and conscious desires cannot be fully known and expressed in prayer without us first coming to know them through the stillness of meditation. Conversely, we won't fully know how to listen for answers in meditation if we have not yet learned how to cast prayer onto our hopes and dreams. As we begin to pray and meditate with some regularity, we will come to intuitively recognize the growth of three positive qualities. First, we will become more compassionate. As we begin to sit in meditation and prayer for longer intervals, we will feel the space around our hearts start to loosen and our love for all beings increase. Further, as we learn how to direct intentions of goodwill to all life, our practice will enable us to act with greater compassion in our day-to-day lives. In fact, a deep and persistent yearning to devote our time to serving all sentient beings will come to nag at our evolving souls.

Through prayer and meditation, we also cultivate a deeper faith in the natural way of things. When we still our minds and open our hearts, a vast world of inner knowing is revealed. This inner space of serenity bursts forth into our consciousness to command more focused attention. As we tap into this sacred space, all events and happenings on the physical plane of reality are imbued with a deeper sense of meaning, purpose, and understanding. Suffering through sickness and disease, landing in prison, being trapped in an abusive relationship, losing a home or job, and experiencing the loss of a loved one are all trying life experiences. Praying and meditating affords us the experience of being present with that kind of intense suffering. And the ability to be present with it offers fresh perspectives from which we can view our own suffering.

Pushing nothing away, we can simultaneously confront the profound emotions of sadness and despair, while gaining deeper insight into the reasons, lessons, and potential for growth that arise from our suffering. The ability to be present, while keeping our hearts open in hell, lifts us into the higher realms of conscious action and brings us into union with the mind of God. Faith is the direct outcome of this communion. As we pray and meditate with greater frequency, a third quality will begin to emerge: an absolute sense of clarity as to the interrelation of all things in the Universe. Within the depths of prayer and meditation, we can't help but feel a deep kinship with all beings of Earth. It is this profound sense of interconnection that sparks monumental shifts in consciousness.

Two Stories, One Heart

When the most recent pandemic hit, an already serious mental health crisis substantially worsened across both the nation and the world. Indicators of this crisis (at least in the United States) included dramatic spikes in suicides, drug overdoses, alcohol abuse, and incidences of domestic violence. These observable indicators were further supported by the fact that a record number of Americans reported gong on anti-anxiety medications and anti-depressants to cope with overwhelming feelings of isolation, sadness, and despair. Several people I spoke to opened up to me about the very real and serious mental health struggles that they faced during the lockdowns and how prayer became their refuge in the face of such enormous suffering.

For example, Sandy D., an elementary school teacher from Kentucky, told me about the crippling anxiety, fear, and depression that she herself felt and saw in her students:

I have been a sixth-grade teacher for fifteen years. But no amount of experience in the classroom could have prepared me for what I witnessed during the pandemic. I saw numerous children break down in the middle of class crying and acting out at frequencies that I had never seen before. I even witnessed two instances of students trying to cut themselves with scissors. [18]

Sandy went on to explain that while it broke her heart to witness the emotional devastation that the period of quarantining caused for her students, the crippling fear and anxiety that she too experienced during that difficult time also began to take a serious toll on her own mental health:

For months on end, the first thing I would do when I signed off from virtual classes or returned home from school (when we returned to face-to-face teaching) was drink large amounts of liquor to cope with the desperation I felt in seeing the utter devastation caused to my students. Eventually, my very supportive and loving husband convinced me to take a year off from work and check into a 4–month alternative alcohol and drug treatment center. It was there at that facility where a real miracle happened in my life. While in residence there, I learned two life-changing spiritual practices that helped me cope with extreme stress and anxiety. First, I learned to place my faith in a higher power through the recitation of daily prayers and affirmations. And then, I was also taught how to meditate. Since taking up both practices, my heart has begun to heal and my own personal resolve in moments of extreme adversity has been strengthened. Today, I am happy to report that I no longer consume even a drop of alcohol. [19]

Sandy was far from the only person I spoke to who took refuge in the sublime healing power of prayer and meditation during the pandemic. Raphael C., a Lyft™ driver and artist from New York City, shared his own personal tale of struggle and how meditation helped him find meaning — and most importantly, gave him the will to live:

When the pandemic happened, I, like many workers in the city's gig economy, suddenly found myself out of work. With far more time on my hands than ever before and with my basic provisions being provided through beefed up unemployment aid, I began to settle into a life in quarantine. But as anyone living in any major city during that time knows, the pandemic wreaked havoc on mental health. I was single at the time of the first round of lockdowns and the crushing alienation from my friends and family led me down into a deep spiral of depression. I remember spending twelve to fifteen hours a day alone in my apartment desperate for human connection. Eventually, that feeling of isolation got so bad that I seriously began to contemplate committing suicide. I came so close to taking my own life that I meticulously planned every detail of how I would do so right down to the exact day and time. [20]

Raphael then went on to share how two days before he had decided to commit suicide, he had a chance encounter with a woman in front of a grocery store who completely revitalized his own faith:

I was walking down the street from my apartment to get something to eat when I encountered a middle-aged Indian woman standing in front of a small neighborhood grocer. As I approached the store, we made immediate eye contact and all I can say is that the look in her eyes communicated to me that she was not living in fear of the pandemic. I felt compelled to stop and talk to her before entering the store. So, I took off my face mask and introduced myself to her. The woman smiled at me and without saying a word pulled out a pocket-sized copy of the Bhagavad Gita (an Indian holy text) from her pocket and handed it to me without any fanfare. In that moment, that is the one thing that stood out to me. She didn't so much as say, "You should read this." She just smiled, handed me the book, and quickly told me her name. And then she just simply said, "I think that both of our work is done for today." She then smiled again and walked away. I still think about that mysterious encounter every day. I don't know, I like to think that maybe she was my guardian angel. Anyways, when I got home that evening I began to flip through the pages of that holy book, and I came upon a passage where Krishna instructs Arjuna on how to meditate. And that was my first introduction to a practice that I began doing every morning and evening during the rest of the lockdowns. In fact, I began to re-perceive that entire lockdown period from one of bitter social isolation to the perfect environment to dive deep into spiritual practice. I credit both that mysterious woman and the practice of meditation with not only saving my life but healing my soul. [21]

Incredibly, not long after our conversation, Raphael revealed to me that he is now enrolled in yoga teacher training and dreams of teaching it to those who suffered like him.

A World in Need of Loving Kindness

Two of the primary purposes of meditation and prayer are learning to let go through cultivating inner faith and becoming aware of our relationship with everything in creation. During periods of crisis like the kind we collectively experienced, metta practice is a fantastic meditation exercise that at once achieves both goals. Metta roughly translates to "benevolence" or "loving kindness" in Pali and comes to us from the Buddhist tradition. The purpose of this practice is to focus on cultivating and sending feelings of goodwill to all sentient beings. I was first introduced to this practice at the first group meditation I ever attended a long time ago. The session was led by a wonderful man named Dave Smith, a highly accomplished teacher in the Theravada tradition. Dave, who has made it his life's work to aid in the recovery of those suffering from substance abuse, led us through a twenty-minute metta practice. In that first sitting, we were asked to imagine sending rays of love from our hearts to all of humanity. This guided meditation so moved my spirit and opened my heart that I began attending Dave's Sunday evening session every week.

Looking back now on that fateful day in early 2013, I am amazed at how completely this simple, yet meaningful practice touched my soul. After years of reflection on the power of the practice, I have come to realize why it is so impactful: loving kindness meditations simultaneously quiet our restless minds and open our wayward hearts. In chaotic and uncertain times, what could be more important than sending our deepest wishes of love and goodwill to the planet when we wake up each morning and go to bed each night? Through the ages, it has been said by more than a few sages that meditation is the highest form of prayer because it breaks down the separation between the external world and our own vast inner world. When love meets prayerful intentions, the possibilities for the evolution of human consciousness are boundless. I have personally witnessed firsthand just how true this is.

Back in my days as a college professor, I made a habit of facilitating meditation gatherings at each of the schools I taught at. As you might imagine, creating such spaces for inner reflection were commonly met with numerous eye rolls as academics are conditioned to worship the thinking mind and dismiss anything else that hints at the existence of an eternal reality beyond the bounds of conceptual thought. However, at each of the schools where these gatherings took place, I noticed something beautiful that emerged among both the students and faculty who regularly attended those weekly one-hour events: a hunger to connect to something deeper than themselves. In those gatherings, I introduced participants to every kind of prayerful meditation imaginable. We did breathwork, recited mantras, engaged in walking meditation, and even chanted together.

However, of all the forms of meditation, loving kindness was the one practice that consistently moved all those in attendance. My favorite metta-adapted exercise was to begin by having those gathered imagine one being who they dearly loved. That being could be a person, a beloved pet, or even a loved one who had passed on. I then instructed them to imagine sending rays of golden light directly from their own hearts to the hearts of the beings they recalled. As they did so, I then had them repeat the following mantra: "I send you love, I send you goodwill, and I send you peace." Next, I would have the participants think of a person with whom they had endured a falling-out. I then instructed them to imagine sending that same golden light from their own hearts to the hearts of that person. As they did so (this part of the exercise proved difficult for many at first) I had them repeat the same mantra: "I send you love, I send you goodwill, I send you peace." However, I then instructed them to add two extra lines at the end of that mantra: "I send you forgiveness and I send you and I both healing." I would then close the exercise by having them imagine sending that same and ever-expansive golden light to everyone gathered in the room, to everyone on campus, to everyone in their community, to everyone in the country — and finally, to all sentient beings everywhere in the world. We would then close the meditation and sit together in silence for a couple minutes.

In the moments following that adapted loving kindness practice, I always felt a heightened energy in the room that at times emitted such powerful vibrations that it gave me goosebumps. On multiple occasions, I remember how some participants burst into tears that seemed to transcend all human emotions. Yet at the same time, I felt an expression of gratitude emanating from them at having been released (if only for a moment) from the suffocating grip of the ego that emphasizes our separateness. It was only after guiding such prayer-filled meditations that I truly began to understand that loving kindness cannot only figuratively heal the world but quite literally as well. When I think back on the power of those gatherings, I can't help but be reminded again of the power expressed when two or more people gather with their prayer intentions focused on love. The meaning of this scriptural verse from Matthew 18:19–20 (in the New Testament) in which Jesus instructs his disciples with these words, "For where two or three gather in my name, there am I with them," perfectly captures the union of pure spirit and love that I felt during those gatherings.

Looking back at our shared experience during that period of adversity, it is crystal clear that the world is in desperate need of more loving kindness and compassion. This is an important lesson that we can take with us moving forward when we inevitably confront another moment of crisis. Regardless of the hand that humanity is dealt with in the future, it is imperative that we all engage in inner work to avoid falling down the cliff of separation again.

Maintaining Prayerful Connections in Times of Crisis

All of the above begs the following question: If prayer and meditation has the kind of immense healing power that helps us grow in our consciousness, how can we stay connected in Spirit through both practices when dramatic events like a public health crisis call for us to be more distant and isolated from one another?

Max Reif, a wise and fantastic voice for the conscious writing collective, The Mindful Word, may have an answer to how we can all stay connected in soulful prayer. In one of his many thoughtful pieces written during the height of the lockdowns, Max (a seeker who I have established a heartfelt connection with over the years through our respective contributions to the publication) shared his experience of how he stayed connected in Spirit to others through virtual interface programs like Zoom™. Throughout that time, his daily meditative routine was inspiring, to say the least:

> I rise, as often as possible, at 5:00 a.m. At 6:30 a.m., I attend "Virtual Morning Arti," an international Zoom™ gathering of Meher Baba devotees. We recite prayers, sing two spiritual anthems, and then spend an hour sharing whatever songs, poems, messages, or anecdotes people are inspired to contribute. This event often leads me to great heights of joy! While the external world continues its hard slog, my internal world is brought to a point of *shining* — more than before the pandemic, I think. [22]

I can personally relate to Max's experience of finding spiritual connection through an online community of seekers in just such a crisis. During the lockdowns, I found myself on a podcast radio tour in promotion of the first edition of this book. Throughout that tour, I was blessed to have been invited as a guest on shows with hip-sounding names like Zen Commuter, Everyday Peace, and Healing from Within. During that five-month-long virtual tour, I met so many wonderful hosts who all shared one thing in common: a genuine desire to inspire others through sharing the light of truth and awakening. Though all the interviews I participated in were done virtually, the depth and quality of those interactions ran so deep that at times I felt as though I had known the hosts for years even though we had just met moments before the show.

Like Max, I found an authentic connection with a cast of characters that I otherwise would not have met had the pandemic never occurred. There were two especially profound moments from those fifty interviews that still stand out in my mind. The first took place at the beginning of one show, when the host, sensing my frazzled energy from the day (this was an evening show), invited me to join her in an unforgettable mindfulness meditation that at once brought grounding to the moment and soothed my ailing heart from a day of highly contentious interactions with colleagues. The comic irony of having been led through a meditation was not lost on me! There I was with my new book, supposed wisdom, and important message to deliver to viewers to "help them." And yet, here was the host calming me down in front of thousands of viewers so that I could get out of my own head and be a clearer channel of awareness. After the interview I remember wondering, *Who was really helping whom?* It was one of those moments that really checked my ego and reaffirmed how attached to my role as a "teacher" I had become. The guided meditation with the host was also so exquisitely lighthearted and beautiful that it made me appreciate once again just how powerful the practice is in helping us find our center.

The other poignant moment from that tour was when a listener called in to our live broadcast to share a story of the tremendous suffering she had endured during the contagion. That caller went on to describe how her husband had very suddenly fallen sick and died and how grief-stricken she was at having lost her partner after thirty happy years of marriage. Tears were rolling down my eyes as I listened to her story. When she was finished speaking all I could muster in reply was my sincere condolences. In that moment I remember thinking that whatever I said would bring very little comfort to her. I also thought that maybe all she really needed was a spark of shared connection and a confirmation that we understood what she was going through. As if reading my thoughts, the host of the show (who was a retired reverend himself) did something quite remarkable. He offered to lead us in a deeply moving prayer for the alleviation of the woman's suffering.

So, there we were — the three of us and a couple thousand listeners — all sharing in prayer from our different locations across the country. Looking back now, I sincerely believe that each one of us (the listeners included) wound up tasting a piece of the healing fruit offered to the caller that day. While I will always prefer the soulfulness of face-to-face interactions of this kind, that moment came as close to any that I've experienced to being a genuine moment of spiritual connection. What I took away from this experience is that the profound healing power of prayer not only transcends time and space, but it is always our inner refuge. This is especially true in times of crisis.

Chapter Six Key Takeaways

- Prayer and meditation are two powerful channels through which we can heal ourselves from within.

- Prayer can be thought of as an invocation or an act of direct communion in which we share our faithful intentions and conscious desires with God, the Universe, the One.

- Meditation is the act of stilling your mind and tuning your soul toward the wisdom of God, the Universe, the One.

- One of the most profound benefits of prayer and meditation is that both spiritual practices allow us to be present with our suffering.

- The most recent pandemic wreaked havoc on our mental health and revealed how much we need to engage in practices like prayer and meditation to help us both relate to and transcend our own suffering.

- It also revealed just how in need the world is of more loving kindness and how loving kindness practices like the Buddhist metta meditation can help alleviate our suffering.

- The Buddhist metta practice is essentially a prayer of peace and goodwill that is extended to all sentient beings.

- The public health crisis also revealed that we don't necessarily have to be face to face to practice and receive the benefits of both prayer and meditation. We can just as easily receive the healing properties of both through participating in conscious online or virtual communities. In other words, the profound healing power of prayer and meditation transcends both time and space.

Chapter Six Meditation

Find a comfortable position seated either upright or with legs crossed. Now close your eyes and tune into your breath. Breathe in and breathe out. As you inhale and exhale, think of someone you know who needs love and healing. Now bring an image of that person to your mind and imagine sending a healing golden light directly from your own heart to theirs. Now picture that golden light being received and spreading through every crevice of the person's body as waves of healing love. Continue transferring this golden light energy while you repeat the following mantra silently to yourself: "I send you light, I send you peace, I send you healing." Now, try to bring your mind to a being who you feel has wronged you or with whom you have (or have had) conflict. No matter how painful or uncomfortable it may be, hold an image of that person in your mind as you repeat the same process of sending golden light from your own heart directly to theirs. As you do so, repeat again this mantra: "I send you light, I send you peace, I send you healing." Now, begin to direct this healing golden light to anyone else who may be in your house or apartment with you. Parents, friends, lovers, pets. Extend this golden light to them and repeat the mantra again: "I send you light, I send you peace, I send you healing." If you live alone without any human or pet companions, direct this healing light to the enlightened beings on your puja table or altar. If you don't presently have either erected, send that light to a guru or other enlightened being. Now, continue to gradually extend that light to people in your neighborhood, community, county, state, nation, and finally, imagine the radiant golden light both circling and permeating the entire world as you sit in outer space looking down at the glorious planet that you and billions of other beings call home. Finally, end the meditation by sending this golden light to yourself while you repeat these words: "I send myself light, I send myself peace, I send myself healing." Now open your eyes, take a few deep breaths, and rest in knowing that your heart and soul has been healed through the power of prayer.

OM.

SEVEN
Earth Communication

A Letter from Earth to Humanity

AT **the height** of the lockdowns, I sat down and wrote the following letter to Earth. I have a feeling that many might relate to the sentiments expressed here...

Dear Humanity,

Earth here. Remember me? This is your eternal mother who feeds you, quenches your thirst, and gives you this gift of life. It has been a long time since I last wrote to you, but I feel obliged to share my thoughts amid the crisis you currently face.

First, let me say that I'm truly sorry for the heavy loss of life that you've endured. Sadly, your megalomaniac rulers are mostly to blame for those who died. In truth, if your systems of power had only cared about the poor, elderly, and most vulnerable in society all along, many more lives could've been saved. However, your authorities have insisted on prioritizing this illusionary thing you call money over the well-being of all of Earth's inhabitants. Greed and a lack of reverence for life is a creed that only results in mass suffering. The great prophets of all your religious traditions taught as much. This all brings me to my main point for writing you this letter: to inspire reflection and hope about the sanctity of your relationship with me. Now that you are stuck at home and forced to sit still for a minute, I figured right now is as good a time as ever to level with you straight!

Please know that I give you everything you need to thrive and flourish. I give you plentiful food and water, rarefied air to fill your lungs with, majestic mountains to climb and gain perspective upon, crystal-clear lakes and rivers to bathe in, beautiful animals to bond with, and even visionary plants to heal and enlighten you. In short, your species is just one tiny fragment of my infinite consciousness. Without me, there is no you. We're not separate, but one.

Please also know that when you build structures that wind up harming me, you're only harming yourself. It's my dharma, my divine duty, to protect all that is holy. So, when your species harms my being, I'm obligated to destroy those very structures in return. This event has painfully revealed how unwisely your species has been living. A truly civilized people teach and live by the values of peace, unity, and love. A truly civilized people also realize their inherent unity with Earth and would never do me harm. Based on your current actions, it appears that your political leaders and captains of industry show little care for the fate of our planet. Massive deforestation, oil and nuclear spills, the widespread contamination of rivers, lakes, and oceans, as well as the mass extinction of precious ecosystems are just a sample of how your worship of consumerism has desecrated my body and spirit.

I hope this crisis has provided a moment of valuable introspection for you. For in the wake of the shutdown of your industries, I began to heal. Did you know that for a brief period, many gathered in the urban centers of India could begin to see my glorious snow-capped peaks for the first time in over half a century?!?! And in that strange land of sensory overload where all your Hollywood actors reside, the smog began to lift, and I could breathe again! I can't begin to describe how great it felt to have this respite from your rampant development schemes! My children, it felt so nice to be released from your suffocating grip of industry!

Now, as I hope many have realized during this time, there exists a path that will bring you eternal peace, harmony, and union with me. The sacred and time-honored traditions of your indigenous peoples hold the secrets to both your future happiness and survival. No matter where or when my beloved guardians have emerged, they've all shared these three things in common:

1. A deep and lived inborn belief that Earth is sacred and is the supreme source of all revelatory wisdom.
2. Established lifestyles in which humans take only the bare minimum of resources they need from me to survive.
3. A long and hallowed commitment to defend me from the onslaughts of society's plunderers.

You now find yourself at a very perilous crossroads. At this moment, you so desperately NEED the wisdom of your indigenous peoples, but sadly you've destroyed the very foundations of their cultures. Rather than honor these faithful devotees of Earth, you insist on desecrating their sacred lands and converting them to your misguided industrial creed. Can't you see that you have relegated these proud cultures to a life of deprivation and detachment from their Earth-honoring traditions? If you are to survive as a species (because if you continue to desecrate me, I will regretfully be forced to defend myself and remove you from the equation), I would strongly recommend that you begin honoring and learning from those people. For my passionate Earth guardians hold the secrets to maintaining eternal balance with me.

I wish to end this letter with a positive and uplifting message. It's never too late to change your ways. If humanity decides to heed these words, then the balance of Earth can be restored and my dream of an everlasting union with you can be realized. Know that I'm pulling for you to succeed. For if you succeed, we both succeed. The choice is yours. Use your gift of free will wisely!

With blessings and love,
Your Earth Mother

The Divinity in Nature

As the Creator humbles, so does the natural world. Who among us can say that they don't feel inconsequential when standing on top of a mountain? It is impossible not to. Anyone who has made the pilgrimage up one reports feeling profoundly humbled. For on the amazing peaks, our souls are moved by the sheer majesty of views that await us: a gorgeous colossus of trees, the mesmerizing stature of nearby summits, the noble presence of soaring eagles, and those subtle but dazzling flashes of white light that sparkle against the backdrop of our great Sun. As we inhale a deep breath of the crisp mountain air, we become instantly aware of our own insignificance in relationship to the Universe. In so doing, we come to (consciously or unconsciously) embrace the notion that humanity is but one tiny wave in a vast sea of oneness.

It is from Mother Nature's power to humble when we uncover the source of pure inspiration. We tap into this coveted but sacred energy through Earth's reservoirs of natural beauty. When we decide to descend back down the same mountain top, we carry this feeling of renewal back with us and inject it into our day-to-day lives. When we feel humbled and inspired by nature, we are in open acknowledgment of her beauty. This is also to say that our souls recognize the presence of God within her being. As beauty is in the eye of the beholder, it can emerge through countless forms in nature like a majestic sunset over the ocean, an enchanting waterfall, red rock formations in the desert, and of course...a breathtaking view from atop a mountain.

The acknowledgment of nature's beauty does not need to be restricted to spectacular sights alone. Indeed, we can encounter it through each of our five physical senses. We may find great beauty in the sweet calls of chirping songbirds or in the refreshing smells that follow an afternoon storm. And as we come to encounter nature's beauty repeatedly over time, we begin to see her perfection expressed through all acts of Earth's creation: from the blossoming of a flower to the owl's evening calls, and even extending to the mystical in-between hour of each day, when it is no longer day and not yet night. Through such sustained and soulful interactions with the natural world, we come to acknowledge her beauty more and more fully. In so doing, we bring ourselves ever closer to the eye of Creation. For what is nature but a mirror reflection of God? Through our communion with Earth, all dualities dissolve into a mountain mist. There is no sense of separation, only the infinite presence of oneness. Within this experience, the Creator's imprints are seen as inexorably ingrained within the earthy particles of creation.

The strong emotions that oneness inspires emerge from the depths of our being. From nature we learn that there is no such thing as the separate self. We are all extensions of Earth. In turn, this direct experience of oneness sparks profound feelings of inner peace. The feelings of peace that are encountered in nature should be familiar to anyone who has walked through the woods or swam in a lake, river, or ocean. It first presents itself as a great stillness. Freed from the endless static and noise of society (particularly in the cities), we are overcome by the air of serenity that reigns in the green oasis. When we take a stroll through the forest, we are struck by the diversity of life that we encounter. Hopping frogs, blissful squirrels, melodic songbirds, budding flowers, and gentle-flowing streams all spark these feelings of serenity. As we begin to find our refuge of peace in nature, the floodgates of freedom are also opened.

However, this freedom is unlike the illusionary kind that we encounter in society. The liberty that we find in the wild cannot be granted nor stripped away by any man-made authority, entity, or institution. It is akin to a type of natural freedom. This type of liberty extends beyond humans to the sacredness of nature. There is no need for any government to safeguard or administer this freedom because the laws of nature supersede any decrees put forth by man. In this sense, freedom is expressed as a family of deer prancing effortlessly through the woods, or as water flowing down a nearby stream. The herds of buffalo, who steadfastly roam the fertile grounds of their ancestors, are another illustration of this sort of liberty. As these images convey, freedom is the soul's unbounded expression of its being. Through the acts of prancing, flowing, and roaming, each derive meaning from what it means to truly be. They are free. And because nature-beings are the living embodiment of freedom in earthly form, they instruct us in what its true components are: independence, spontaneity, free will, clarity of purpose, and courage.

Beings in the wild are independent in the sense that they provide for their own sustenance, determine (for the most part) when it is time to hunt for prey, are unfettered by the absence of playing cultured roles, have relative control over where they roam and settle, and are not beholden to future expectations put upon them. Above all, nature-beings do not consciously impede upon the free will of others to act. They respect the natural state of independence that all beings in the wild have. The coyote does not place burdensome restrictions on the chipmunks. It does not require them to give up half of all their stored nuts for winter hibernation in exchange for it not eating them. Nor does the strongest chimpanzee male conjure up malicious schemes to swindle the rest of the pack out of their share of the hunting booty. For if he did so, that alpha would be swiftly and violently replaced! Similarly, the bear does not proselytize to the deer. It stays clear from dictating matters of divinity. The bear lives IT instead. Nature, then, is eternal truth. For there are no facades, deceptions, or falsehoods in the purity of the wild. The trees do not dress up in business suits to convince the river to purchase its fallen leaves. Nor does the mountain flash a plastic smile to coax the valley into submitting to its rule.

Deep within, each of us *know* that nature is the truth. Despite the many distractions that man creates for itself, our greatest joys are experienced through communing with Earth. In fact, this feeling of contentment is so intrinsic, that many people dream of one day acquiring enough money to retire away to a body of water or to the mountains. This intuitive drive to connect with our mother never wavers. Not even for those of us living in the Western world, where alienation from nature is most severe. As we come to honor this innate drive to connect with Earth, we will all notice the existence of divine qualities in the wild. For example, trees embody the resolute and formidable statue of God in form. They also reflect ITs exquisite wisdom through their enduring presence and faith in the natural cycles of rain and sun. Likewise, the mountains capture the mystical heights of the Highest through its power to convey perspective.

Perhaps there is no clearer representation of divinity in nature than the Sun. The Sun is the essence of creation. Besides providing for Earth's sustenance, it is also our spiritual guide and mentor. For the Sun's rays permeate the depths of our souls with its life-giving compassion. Yet, even as the Sun makes our existence possible, it derives something just as meaningful in return: the fulfillment of its own purpose. So, even as the Sun nourishes life, its own infinite spirit is uplifted through the gift of sharing in the mysterious wonder of this creation. In short, Earth is our purest and most abundant source of divine connection.

Reforging a Bond with the Wild

Often I wonder why people feel obliged to build structures to connect with the Divine when that connection can most easily and innately be felt while gardening, swimming in a lake, or hiking through the forest. Whenever people ask me how they can better connect with the truth of living Spirit, one of the first things I tell them is to strap on their boots and commune with Earth. For she is the very source of that living Spirit.

During the most recent pandemic, an interesting phenomenon took place. Countless people began moving from large, densely populated cities to suburbs and smaller communities in the rural countryside. The growing popularity of remote work, strict lockdowns in urban areas, and fear of catching the virus all contributed to this occurrence. But one often overlooked reason for that reverse migration of sorts from urban to rural areas, which also had a lot to do with our deep yearning to live in closer proximity to nature. It served as a wake-up call that our culture's alienation from the natural world has had grave consequences for our mental, physical, and spiritual health. For many people living in big cities, the lockdowns proved unbearable. And for some, like Kevin S., a tech worker from Philadelphia, Pennsylvania, the mental anguish they caused became a catalyst to move away from the city and closer to nature:

> For a time, the lockdowns in Philly were just unbearable in terms of the social isolation I felt. But during that challenging time, I found myself thinking about the Rocky Mountains multiple times a day. While my physical body was trapped in the confines of the city, my mind and spirit were in the mountains. It had always been a dream of mine to live in Montana. I fondly remember taking a visit out there with my father when I was a teenager and just feeling blown away by the snow-capped peaks and visiting the spectacular Glacier National Park. Ever since that trip, I made a vow to myself that I would move there at some point in my life. [23]

Kevin went on to add:

I had grown up in a rural part of Pennsylvania and I went to college there as well. But after graduating, I decided to move to Philly in search of a high-paying job, a top-notch music scene, and of course, to meet people from many walks of life. But late at night, while lying in bed in my overcrowded apartment complex, I would think about that trip I took with my father up to Montana and hiking several peaks. But it took the pandemic to make me realize how much I desperately needed to leave the city and move out to Montana to reconnect with nature. After the lockdowns ended, I packed up my bags and moved to White Fish, Montana to live out my dreams. [24]

Taylor R., a hospitality worker from Boston, Massachusetts, expressed some similar sentiments as Kevin S. about her desire to reconnect with nature during the lockdowns:

When the pandemic hit, I lost my job at a high-end hotel bar. During my time away from work, I realized that I was presented with a perfect opportunity to move nearer to nature. So, I moved across country to California just outside Yosemite National Park. I can't describe the peace I have felt since moving here. That whole public health scare really put things in perspective for me and made me acknowledge how central to my life Earth should be. [25]

We are living in an age of unprecedented comfort, convenience, and technological advancement. Yet, despite all the assurances from our cultural leaders and institutions that we are living the "good life" with all our economic prosperity and consumerism, deep down we know that something is off. We are detached from the natural world. During the lockdowns, we had ample time to reflect while quarantining in our houses and that led many of us to begin looking inward for guidance. In our meditations, one of the first things we discovered was that reforging a bond with Earth is as natural as breathing or drinking water. And so, some of us started a garden, while others began going on frequent walks through the woods to connect with the spirit of our Earth mother. Still, others went to even greater lengths to connect with the wild.

In that tumultuous time, I can vividly remember an instance when an extremely bright past student of mine suddenly stopped showing up to classes and instead set off on a cross-country journey with only this one goal in mind: to visit every major national park in the country. The Colorado Rockies, the Grand Tetons, Olympic National Forest, Joshua Tree, the Grand Canyon, Yellowstone — you name it — and he visited there while braving storms and camping out under the stars. To this day, I truly believe his time was much better spent pursuing that inspiring goal than had he remained in my own class! What he accomplished is what I would call a first-rate education. Clearly, a sincere yearning to connect with Earth was present in that young man's heart. And who could help but admire that young man's courage to embark on such an epic journey in the middle of an otherwise terrifying event for so many? The point of that story is that our innate desire to connect with Earth can only be suppressed for so long. During the earliest days of the lockdowns, I received this fitting email from an elderly woman named Carol in response to a piece I wrote about how that event reawakened our love of nature:

> Isn't it interesting to hear the silence again? No cars on the road spewing their harmful emissions in the air! The streets are quiet, but the parks are full of people who are maybe realizing once more that we are not separate from Earth. I don't wish this virus on anyone but hearing the sounds of the birds chirping again is just oh so sweet. [26]

The Sacred Covenant

Clearly, one lesson that was imparted to all of us during the pandemic was how important nature is to our lives. It should go without saying then, that staving off the ecological catastrophe (already underway) requires all of us to restore what I like to call a sacred covenant with Earth. But what does such a covenant entail? The first part of this covenant demands that we treat her in the same way that we would a beloved partner, family member, or pet — with dignity and respect. What is needed is for us not to take more than we need from her to survive and to cease our senseless exploitation of her precious resources (big oil executives, I am staring at you!).

The second part of this covenant implies that we resolve to learn and honor the ways of our indigenous peoples who for countless millennium have maintained an exquisite balance in living symbiotically with Earth. On this point, I have had the privilege of deepening my friendship with a beloved Cherokee elder named Myrtle Driver. And what I have learned from visiting this selfless preserver of the Cherokee language and servant of her people is that much of their culture's way of life revolves around honoring the sacredness of nature. Engaging in deliberate practices that desecrate our mother is simply unfathomable to the teachings of all indigenous traditions. It is imperative then, that we here in the West work to preserve those very cultures that hold the wisdom in how to live with ecological awareness and balance. To destroy our indigenous cultures is literally like severing a tree from its roots.

The third part of this covenant requires that we each make a concerted daily effort (if possible) to connect with Earth in some way. This could be as simple as planting a small garden or taking a short thirty-minute walk on the coastline, in the mountains, or at the city park. However we choose to connect is up to each of us individually. I have come to believe that when we each develop an intimate connection with Earth, we become more likely to stand up and protect her from would-be human predators. Would you stand by if someone threatened to harm your beloved partner, friend, or pet? Absolutely not. Our intimate relationship with Earth should breed that same kind of loyalty that we extend to our loved ones.

Finally, the fourth part of this covenant calls on all of us to become "nature missionaries." This means that we each play a role in exposing others to nature. Among my own group of friends, one of the things I am known for (other than being that hippie guy who is always running late!) is taking people out on hikes in the mountains where I live. I can't count how many times I have led "nature newbies" on hikes and witnessed their joy in communing with the wonders of the natural world...sometimes for the first time. The feeling I get from seeing the awe on their faces when experiencing a mesmerizing sunset or dramatic view is priceless. Nature feeds our souls. And when our souls are fed in that way, we can't help but become passionate advocates and protectors of Earth ourselves.

We are all keepers of this sacred covenant. And we all receive our spiritual nourishment from honoring her with every ounce of our being. Earth is our greatest source of wisdom, connection, and love.

Chapter Seven Key Takeaways

- The qualities of the natural world reflect the Divine. The beauty, wonder, and peace that Earth inspires is a direct manifestation of the Highest.

- Our connection to Earth is sacred.

- The most recent pandemic provided a valuable opportunity for us all to reflect on our own relationship with nature.

- Through such spirited self-reflection, many of us discovered that we were not in fact honoring this sacred relationship and that the consequences of not doing so has brought us out of balance emotionally, physically, and spiritually.

- In response to the isolation experienced during the lockdowns, many of us chose to move away from highly dense urban areas to the countryside.

- A deep yearning to connect with nature is innate within all of us and was, in fact, a major factor for many people in deciding to move away from the cities.

- The profound importance of establishing a sacred covenant with nature is perhaps one of our greatest takeaways from that time.

- This sacred covenant has four parts. First, we must honor and care for Earth in the same way that we honor and care for a beloved partner, family member, or pet. Second, we must resolve to learn and honor the ways of our indigenous peoples who for countless millennium have maintained an exquisite balance in living symbiotically with Earth. Third, we must each make a concerted daily effort (if possible) to connect with Earth in some way. Finally, we must become "nature missionaries," meaning that we each actively seek to expose others to the healing power of the natural world.

Chapter Seven Meditation

Set aside a couple hours for a slow and meditative walk in nature. As you begin your walk, immerse yourself in the majesty of nature and observe the stunning combination of beauty, truth, wonder, and balance in the wild. Observe the miraculous happenings of Earth. The delightful sounds of birds singing their heartfelt songs... Roaring creeks ebbing and flowing as an eternal expression of absolute being... Golden leaves falling from ancient trees as playful squirrels collect their nuts for winter. Take a moment to breathe in the crisp cool air as you meander along and ponder the evolution of sacred Earth who sustains you. She is infinitively older than you can possibly fathom. And she is infinitely wiser than you can ever comprehend. Revel in the sublime wonder of how all her diverse features form one picture-perfect mosaic. Continue to take note of sights, sounds, and smells. Then experience the ecstatic feeling as your soul becomes one with the trees, rocks, soil, and sky. You are one with it all. There exists no separation between you and your own Earth Mother. Any notion of separation is merely an illusion. As you walk, continue bringing your attention to your breath and repeat this mantra to yourself: "I am one with Earth." Repeat it again: "I am one with Earth." Repeat this mantra as many times as necessary until you experience your total unity with her. As you continue repeating your mantra, "I am one with Earth," lie down on your stomach with your face fully down on the ground and your arms extended directly forward. Now kiss Earth three times. With each kiss, imagine Earth filling your heart with love and you returning that love back to her. You are a child of Earth; born from the grace of your mother, and at play with all the plants and animals in the wild. Let your soul run free. Let it merge with Earth's vibrations of stillness.

OM.

EIGHT
Creative Self-Expression

The Wonder of Creativity

ONE day a painting caught my eye as I roamed through an art museum in Nashville, Tennessee. The artwork was a depiction of the inside of a human body. Rather than portray its skeletal features, the artist sketched the energy or chakra points of the being. The body was painted the colors of the primary seven access points and depicted waves of energy (of the same colors) flowing into and out from the body. For an hour straight, I stared at this painting in awe contemplating the state of consciousness that the artist was trying to convey. The message of the painting was clear: at our core we are made of energy and our true essence is not physical but spiritual. If one painting can deliver this truth, then so can one song, photo, or poem. As we each awaken into our being, we start to feel an insatiable desire to share our own inner transformation with others. The soul's vehicle of communication is creative expression. And it takes many forms.

Music might be the most powerful medium of creativity. How many of you have experienced the feelings of pure joy while dancing or performing music? To me, reggae is the genre that absolutely transports me to a state of pure ecstasy. The driving baseline, soulful lyrics, and positive vibrations that reggae delivers sends me into such a state of raptures that I literally feel the need to drag anyone at the show with me onto the dance floor to share in the energy exchange. I have come to believe that music, particularly if musicians use it as a form of worship, is one of the most inspiring forces on the planet for its power to move and unite people across different cultures, ethnicities, and nationalities.

The written word, too, is a profound channel for the soul's expression. After all, some of the most inspiring written works in history have been those about spiritual transcendence. The Bhagavad Gita, the Bible, and the Tao Te Ching are all notable examples, as are more modern visionary works of writing such as Kahlil Gibran's *The Prophet*, Hermann Hesse's *Siddhartha,* and Henry David Thoreau's *Walden.* Poetry, too, is a unique and inspired form of written expression, for it provides a direct pathway into our shared experience of reality. Poetry also conveys in a few short lines what it takes entire books to write. Its brevity reflects its heartfelt sincerity and deep contact with the present moment.

As expressions of living Spirit, we can communicate deeply felt truths through all creative outlets. While sharing our art is intimately personal, it is also paradoxically communal in the sense that it speaks to the unity of our journeys on the path. To me, a world without creative expression would not be a life worth living. In the words of the legendary reggae band, Steel Pulse: "Life, life without music, I can't go." [27] Art, the written word, photography, and even storytelling (one of the oldest modes of creative expression) informs us of the richness of the human experience and allows us to intuitively feel our innate connection to being.

Matthew Fox, a mystic priest and theologian, wrote a beautiful little book called, *Creativity: Where the Divine and Human Meet.* In it, he explores how the highest communion to that living Spirit can be found right at our fingertips in the simplest expressions of human creativity. Further, he suggests that the most prayerful and spiritually powerful act a person can undertake is to create with an awareness of the place from which that gift arises. Fox's ideas are wise because they are true! I suspect that many of you who are reading this now have directly experienced what he is talking about. For when we are absorbed in any creative act, we enter a timeless space and we feel fulfilled. But what exactly is that sense of fulfillment we feel in those gloriously creative moments? That feeling is our soul's revelation of oneness that results from entering a direct communion with the source of Creation. We feel fulfilled because our natural state is one of creative synergy with all that is IT. And when we create out of an awareness of that sacred place from which creativity arises, the power of our creative act is amplified many times over.

I can still remember the first time when I knew that creative expression is a direct gift from God. Many years back, I found myself jamming with a group of very talented musician friends of mine. I was happily playing percussion. At some point in the night, our impromptu jam session took on a life of its own. I recall being so enthralled and overcome by the bliss of playing that at one point I turned to my friend who was on the lead guitar and exclaimed, "This is simply divine and now I fully get why you guys devote your lives to playing music (my friends were in a nationally touring band at the time)." In response to my comment, my friend simply gave me a knowing nod and we kept right on grooving! When the jam session did finally wind down, I distinctly remember looking at my phone and being surprised that it was 2:00 in the morning. We had jammed for five straight hours! IT didn't matter that my hands were raw from hitting the djembe and bongos all night because I had touched a place beyond any sense of mild physical discomfort. I was aware that what I had just experienced was a gift of the One.

Since that memorable jam session, now whenever I sit down to write, play, and perform music or deliver a consciousness-themed talk, I try to take a moment to give thanks to the Creator for that gift of creation. And always, I strive my very best (but of course I do not always succeed) to make my words or music an act of supreme worship. In so doing, I like to offer my creative act as devotion to the Highest. Because in truth, the act of creative self-expression is like Brahman serving Brahman. For the creative act itself is a gift from Brahman, channeled through you, the creative conduit, as a manifestation of Brahman, and shared with others who are also manifestations of Brahman — all to bring everyone, including you, the artist, closer to Brahman in a moment of total love.

The Hippies and the Last Great Renaissance in Art

In times of great adversity, all human beings (whether conscious of this fact or not) are challenged to question the very meaning of their existence. Events such as war, economic collapse, natural disasters, political upheaval, and pandemics have the effect of shaking men and women out of their day-to-day routines and sense of comfort. As history clearly shows, these ages have also sparked some of the most profound and inspiring renaissances in the creative arts. Just as we cannot separate the river's journey from its destination to the vast blue ocean, so can't we separate revolutions in the creative arts from their societal contexts. As a case in point, consider the renaissance of art that took place during the 1960s and 70s.

In a global context, this age had it all. A hugely unpopular and devastating war in Vietnam, the Cold War, the looming threat of nuclear devastation, independence movements around the world, and women's liberation on both sides of the Atlantic. In short, for much of the planet, social revolution and war came to define that period's external landscape. Unquestionably, the escalation of extreme government violence amid a backdrop of mass protests and growing existential fears gave rise to an inspiring movement of higher consciousness that became embodied by the hippie counterculture. At its core, the hippies were at the forefront of a movement that sought to promote a more soulful and natural way of living in harmony with Creation. On the surface, they saw an external world marked by widespread fear, greed, mindless conformity, and hypocrisy. In response to society's madness, the hippies turned inward through such outlets as meditation, experimentation with visionary plants, and communing with nature. This great period of inner searching saw an explosion of raw creativity that simultaneously served as a deep social commentary of the unjust nature of society while also sharing hopeful visions of transcended states of awareness.

The hippies' powerful merging of an outer world critique and an inner vision of untapped hope, peace, and unity found its soulful expression most powerfully through music. Household acts like The Beatles, Bob Marley, Jimi Hendrix, Pink Floyd, Led Zeppelin, The Who, Jefferson Airplane, Janis Joplin, Bob Dylan, Neil Young, The Doors, and the Grateful Dead communicated the hippie ethos through the vehicle of sound. But this era's renaissance in art was not limited to music alone. Beatnik poets and counterculture authors like Allen Ginsberg, Jack Kerouac, William S. Burroughs, Ken Kesey, and Gary Snyder accomplished through words what musicians did through music. And who can fail to mention three of the most impactful consciousness writers of that generation: Baba Ram Dass, Aldous Huxley, and Alan Watts.

Far too often, when mainstream historians write about the hippie counterculture, they place undue influence on the hedonistic elements of that movement which they caption with the now popular and infamous phrase: "sex, drugs, and rock and roll." But what those same historians fail to mention is that the explosion of raw creativity in that time came from an authentically spiritual place. Am I denying that there weren't instances of wild hedonism on display during that era? Absolutely not! Of course, there was. But there are instances of wild hedonism on display in our own current time as well. In fact, you could make an argument that our hedonistic displays are far worse today than it has ever been. In any case, the art renaissance of the hippie era was chiefly an expression of people's inner desire for an ascended state of consciousness. This same desire to transcend our egos is just now beginning to find expression once more.

Into a New Age of Creativity

In a similar vein as the hippie era, the most recent pandemic primed humanity for the current renaissance of art. Many decades from now, when we look back on that period, we may even come to find that the latest art resurgence eclipsed the creative genius of the 1960s counterculture. There is no doubt that our collective experience provided the ultimate context and fuel for a tidal wave of creativity. While that tumultuous event produced much suffering, it was precisely the experience of it that sparked inner reflection of our own mortality. In truth, it forced much of humanity to confront those questions that define our very existence. Some of these questions are the same ones that have consumed the minds of philosophers and the souls of mystics through time. They include: "Who am I?" "What happens when

I die?" "Will I be reborn?" "What is my purpose here on Earth?" "Who or what is God?" Many beings have felt drawn to the creative arts to express their own answers to these perennial questions.

From my own practice, I can honestly say that I have felt a deeper yearning than ever before to express my admittedly limited understanding to anyone willing to listen. I feel that my own personal experience during the viral outbreak filled me with a greater sense of urgency to convey universal truths through any creative channel available to me. During that time, I wrote the book that you are reading now. I also completed a short story collection about the possibility of transitioning into higher states of awareness. I also began performing live instrumental music and delivered meditation workshops through virtual platforms like Zoom™. These experiences taken collectively finally sparked a recognition within me that I am an artist! The truth is that deep down we are all artists. Do you hear the truth in that? We are all artists. With no exceptions. I have become so sure of this fact, that now whenever I hear someone say to me, "Forrest, I have no artistic talent," my immediate response to that comment is to reply by saying, "You have no artistic talent that you have discovered as of yet." The desire to create and express should feel as natural to us all as talking, breathing, or walking. And if it doesn't feel natural it is not proof that you lack artistic ability. It is merely that you haven't yet opened yourself to that innate drive to create and express.

In the aftermath of the lockdowns, I witnessed this same growing sense of urgency to create and express in many other people as well. Austin Smith, a very talented musician and dear friend of mine who was the lead singer and guitarist of that same nationally touring reggae band I told of jamming with above, described the power of creative expression during the most recent pandemic:

> My personal experience during the pandemic was both challenging and transitional but also fulfilling and enlightening. I spent the last decade leading a national touring band but at the end of 2019 we decided we needed a break from the road and the daily grind of trying to make money with our passion of writing, recording, and performing music. It couldn't have been better timing, as all of us know 2020 was a big change for each of us. One memorable experience during that time was performing concerts for my neighbors from my front porch! Having spent most of my time on the road, these "Quarantine Sessions" became an amazing opportunity to meet and interact with my neighbors for the first time ever. It was a real bright spot of community and togetherness in a dark time of fear and isolation. [28]

The power of creative expression to build "community and togetherness" is something that we humans have long known. Austin's words are proof that in moments of social chaos an artist's urge to express themselves stems from an innate desire to heal humanity. In the wake of that period of lockdowns, I have encountered more creative people than I can ever recall meeting who have adopted ingenious methods to convey the healing message of peace. I have seen street performance art re-emerge and I have participated in more spontaneous music gatherings and drum circles than I can ever recall joining. I have also marveled over the work of transcendent visionary painters who all share an interest in uplifting humanity through their art.

For Diana P., a singer-songwriter from Asheville, North Carolina, the healing power of music was the major factor for why she began busking in the city's downtown during the most recent pandemic:

> I have been playing music all my life. And it has gotten me through some very rough times in my life. You name it — painful breakups, periods of depression, and the deaths of loved ones. So, when the last pandemic happened, I quickly saw that everybody around me was struggling to cope physically, mentally, and emotionally. So, I responded to that event in the only way I knew how: through playing music. For three months straight, every Tuesday and Friday evening I set up downtown and just sang and played my heart out. I didn't receive much in the way of tips when playing but that wasn't at all my motivation. When playing, it warmed my heart to see how much my music uplifted so many people during that difficult time. I literally recall several people walking up to me and just thanking me for making their day better. To me, that reflects the power of music and why I play. [29]

There is another layer to the story of the most recent public health crisis and how that event was a catalyst for this new age of creative self-expression. In their futile attempts to contain that virus, government officials around the world ordered unprecedented shutdowns of several key industries. Their impact had far-reaching and unforeseen consequences for humanity. On the one hand, the massive shutdowns facilitated the full-scale meltdown of the global financial system and led to an unemployment crisis not seen since the height of the Great Depression. Predictably, the shock to the economy also exasperated our collective fear and inflicted significant hardships on many workers and exasperated an already serious mental health crisis. On the other hand, due to subsequent rounds of "social distancing" and home quarantining, most of the world's population found more time for solitude than ever before.

Inevitably, remarkable works of art proved to be one outcome from sustained periods of solitude. While enduring long periods of social isolation can absolutely induce depression and mental health problems among people, it can also spur remarkable works of creative expression in others. In fact, the suffering that we can acknowledge and experience in periods of extended solitude may itself be a muse for the greatest of creative works. Just think for one moment of all the writers, painters, and musicians who have retreated into solitude following painful life events only to remerge weeks, months, or even years later with masterful works of art. The list of these artists contains names too numerous to count.

During the lockdowns, vast injustices within our current political and economic paradigms were dramatically exposed to the world. As the world grappled to cope with the fallout from that event, deep and longstanding societal problems were fully revealed for us all to see...further feeding revivals in art, music, and the written word. That chaotic period in history showed that immoral values like greed and violence currently underlie the foundations of our world. For an entire year, much of humanity literally saw that the emperor had no clothes! And it didn't matter if you were on the right or left of the political spectrum. The deep-seeded political and economic corruption on all sides was stripped bare for all of us to see.

In the years and even decades ahead, we can expect many peaceful souls to do what their forebearers did during the hippie counterculture. The era of a new renaissance in creative expression is upon us. To all artists and creative souls, the time is now to do what you do best: CREATE, MOVE, INSPIRE! Through your art, reveal the absurdity of organizing our societies around the worst aspects of the human condition. But even more important, through your creative acts share the hope that exists in recognizing that death is not to be feared, that love will always prevail, and that we are all one. In periods of shared suffering, the reality of our eternal oneness is easier for all to see. Communicating the truth of our cosmic unity serves the highest and noblest aims of creative expression.

Chapter Eight Key Takeaways

- As we each awaken into our being, we will start to feel an insatiable desire to share our own inner transformation with others.
- The soul's vehicle of communication is creative expression.
- Music, painting, poetry, and photography are all examples of soulful expression that brings us more deeply into the present moment.
- The highest communion with living Spirit can be found right at our fingertips in the simplest expressions of human creativity.
- One of the most prayerful and spiritually powerful acts a person can undertake is to create with an awareness of the place from which the gift of creation itself arises.
- The act of creative self-expression is like Brahman serving Brahman. For the creative act itself is a gift from Brahman, channeled through you, the creative conduit, as a manifestation of Brahman, and shared with others who are also manifestations of Brahman — all to bring everyone, including you, the artist, closer to Brahman in a moment of total love.
- The 1960s hippie counterculture was the last great renaissance in art prior to now.
- In a striking parallel to the hippie era, the most recent pandemic primed humanity for the latest renaissance of art. Many decades from now when we look back on that period, we may even come to find that the latest art resurgence eclipsed the creative genius of the 1960s counterculture.
- For the first time in decades, the period of lockdowns forced us to contemplate the difficult questions that are typically buried beneath our everyday consciousness. Some of these questions are ones that have consumed the minds of philosophers and the souls of mystics through time. They include: "Who am I?" "What happens when I die?" "Will I be reborn?" "What is my purpose here on Earth?" "Who or what is God?" Many beings have felt drawn to the creative arts to express their own answers to these perennial questions.
- During that difficult period, creative expression brought significant comfort and healing to many people.
- In periods of shared suffering, the reality of our eternal oneness is apparent for all to see. Communicating the truth of our cosmic unity serves the highest and noblest aims of creative expression.

Chapter Eight Meditation

To begin this meditation, find a comfortable position either seated upright or with legs crossed. Now, grab a pen and some paper and begin to write a short poem, song lyrics, or a short reflection of no less than six lines and no more than fifteen. You are free to write on whatever theme you want — the only criteria are that your poem, lyrics, or short reflection relate in some way to spiritual reality or to the personal journey of awakening. Here are two examples I wrote:

Example 1:
> Stars align
> Beyond space and time
> A figment of our minds
> Or imaginations?
> Living Spirit resides
> Within the Divine
> Hear it speak through prayer and meditation.

Example 2:
> Awareness flows from Spirit
> Moving nowhere and everywhere
> Beyond the Void
> Producing desires
> That in turn creates our thoughts
> And like the infinite ocean
> Expressing itself as waves
> Our thoughts manifest as intentions
> Spurring us into action
> With mindfulness or not
> As to whether our deeds
> Will harmonize our souls
> With the symphony of the Universe.

As you write, try not to worry about the quality of your poem, song lyrics, or short reflection. For artistic quality is in the eye of the beholder. Instead, just put your pen down on paper and allow your soul to intuitively guide you in the act of creating. Trust that it knows what to do. Now, when you have finished writing, jot down these two questions on the same page just below your creative work — together they will be the focus of this meditation:

Question 1: What deeper meaning were you trying to convey about spiritual reality or the journey of awakening in your writing?

Question 2: Who is it that wrote the poem, song lyrics, or short reflection? In other words, was it you who wrote it? Or rather, did those words derive from a higher power or Source?

As soon as you finish writing down these questions, close your eyes, take three long deep breaths, and quietly contemplate each one of these questions. Mediate on each one of these questions for at least seven to ten minutes. Feel free to set a timer if that helps keep you focused. Whenever it feels right, after that allotted time for contemplation, open your eyes and on the same piece of paper pick up your pen again and write your answers below for both questions. The idea here is not to think too rationally about what came to you during your meditation but to write down what immediately comes to your mind in streams of conscious thoughts. When you have completed the exercise, simply put down your pen and paper and sit quietly for a couple more minutes as you reflect further on the divinity behind every creative act of expression.

OM.

NINE
Self-Sufficiency as a Road to Self-Mastery

The Two Kinds of Self-Sufficiency

IN 1967, before a gathering of youth in San Francisco, CA, Timothy Leary coined a phrase that perfectly captured the mindset of an entire generation. The phrase was, "Turn on, tune in, drop out." In just six words, this counterculture icon powerfully conveyed a message of direct spiritual seeking and non-engagement with the dominant paradigm. If we live by the wisdom of this phrase, we will inevitably find ourselves standing on the outside looking in at society. This reality begs the following question: What is a seeker of truth supposed to do when their consciousness expands so dramatically that compliance with the values, expectations, and norms of their culture are no longer possible?

The answer is that we must become self-sufficient in both thought and action. The thought part means turning your mind to the truth within yourself and not to what is being propagandized on the outside. It means learning to think critically and forming your own thoughts about how to best navigate life and optimize opportunities for self-growth through spirited self-reflection. The action part means engaging in activities with the intention of becoming independent through taking steps like growing your own food, providing for your own and your family's defense, collecting your own rainwater, and finding an alternative energy source to power your own home. It also means working out an independent and workable system of consensus-driven decision making (such as direct democracy) as well as participating in a more local, just, and sustainable economy within our communities. Being truly self-sufficient in both thought and action go hand in hand. The move to become so in action is born from free and independent thought that sees a different way of relating to the world as possible.

Self-Sufficiency in Thought

Back in my days as a college professor, I used to make it a habit of telling my students that they know more than they think they do. I said that to get them to see that intuitive wisdom (as opposed to simple book knowledge) is what they should be after. I would then explain to them how most of life's answers can be found through simply looking within ourselves. Hence the phrase: "You know more than you think you do." I would then explain to them that becoming more critical self-sufficient thinkers serves two positive purposes. First, it makes it less likely that we will fall prey to societal conditioning that aims at pulling us from the source of intuitive wisdom. Second, through looking within for answers we become more self-sufficient in action. I would then tell them the following story:

> A recent high school graduate who was confused about his next step in life went to a very renown life coach in town for a one-time visit. After paying a small fee, the life coach asked the young man what was troubling him. The recent high school graduate then went on to describe how all his high school friends were going to college but that he didn't think it was the path for him. He then expressed his concern to the life coach that he must be a failure for not wanting to follow the traditional path prescribed to him by all his past teachers. A twinkle shined in the eyes of the life coach and a great big smile spread across his face as he extended out his arm to shake hands with the young man. The life coach then exclaimed, "You too feel like a failure for not following the traditional life path? Welcome to the club of free thinkers! If you aim to live an exciting and spiritually enriching life, then this club will bring you great fulfillment. But I must warn you young friend, that it is a lonely club designed for the truly courageous self-sufficient thinker." With a suddenly quiet mind and open heart, the young high school graduate then got up from his seat, thanked the life coach, and strode confidently out of his office and back out into the world with a new sense of purpose. [30]

Now, the punchline to this story is that while his peers were in college, that young high school graduate went on to travel the world volunteering on sustainable farms learning how to become self-sufficient. Today, that grown man now spends much of his time in developing nations in Africa and South America leading workshops on sustainable agriculture to local farmers. I met this most remarkable man at an event that I was speaking at years ago. After sharing his story, the one thing that really stood out to me was how he said that not following the traditional path was a key for him in living an exciting and spiritually enriching life...just as that life coach said it would! If that story doesn't get every college-aged student questioning the reasons and motivations they are there, then what will?

There are several lessons from that story that can easily be applied to our own experiences during the most recent pandemic. Looking back now, I think we could all agree that critical self-sufficient thought was sorely lacking throughout much of that time. Rather than looking within to our own intuitive wisdom, many of us instead turned outside to so-called experts for guidance. One consequence of not consulting our own innate intelligence was that we were herded like hapless sheep into a toxic environment of fear and ignorance. For all the media's emphasis on political division, one irony is that both sides of the spectrum capitalized on our own lack of critical self-sufficient thought to push their own agendas.

Another closely related consequence of not looking within for answers during that period was that we came to embrace extremist beliefs. As discussed before, these beliefs emerged on both ends of the political spectrum. One side projected such fear onto the pandemic that a sizable segment of the population literally supported policies that would be considered totalitarian in normal times such as the mandatory closure of businesses, vaccine mandates, and enforced curfews. And of course, a sizable segment of the population also openly embraced wild conspiracy theories that bordered on sheer madness. The impacts of which severely downplayed the real threat of the contagion to at-risk populations and prevented an early and effective response to it.

Yet a third consequence of not listening to our "still small voice within," to borrow a phrase central to the Quaker religion, is that it temporally relegated our personal faith to the backburner. Simply put, the expressed perspective of people with genuine faith was dismissed. That perspective held that the virus was out of our control and that what was needed was for us to surrender to the moment and to come to the aid of our neighbors and family where we could. People with this faith-based perspective didn't respond to that event with either fear or ignorance. Instead, they allowed themselves to surrender to the suffering that event presented with a clear mind and open heart.

Self-Sufficiency in Action

Stephen Gaskin, the late co-founder of The Farm (founded in 1971), a well-known and remarkable off-the-grid hippie community in Summertown, Tennessee, once said the following about the promise of self-sufficiency in his delightful book, *This Season's People: A Book of Spiritual Teachings:*

> It is revolutionary growing your own food instead of supporting the profit system. It is revolutionary to deliver your own babies instead of paying thousands of dollars a head to profit-oriented hospitals and doctors. It is revolutionary to get the knowledge out of college and make it so you don't have to sell your soul to learn something. It is revolutionary to learn how to fix stuff, rather than junk it or take it in to be replaced. [31]

For Gaskin, The Farm's successful experiment in self-sufficient living was itself a profound expression of opposition to our dependency on society. Unfortunately, in many ways, the most recent pandemic showed us the extent to which most of us are not at all self-sufficient in the ways that Gaskin imagined. Indeed, it showed us just the opposite: just how reliant we are on what might be called the "consumer convenience machine."

Our heavy dependence on the commercial for-profit food system that Gaskin mentions is just one notable example. At multiple points during the most recent pandemic, irrational fear driven by our overdependence led to mass panic shopping in the United States. Back at the start of that event, I can still vividly recall walking through the supermarket in Boulder, Colorado (where I was living at the time) and witnessing the total panic among shoppers as the shelves carrying once fully stocked commodities (such as toilet paper) were completely barren. And I also remember visiting another local market and seeing two separate fights break out between customers over the last carton of eggs. In short, that chaotic event taught us that if you want to witness the breakdown of modern society, just threaten to cut off our food supply chains! In response to all that panic over food and other commodity shortages, I recalled thinking at the time how absurd it was that we are so dependent on a centralized supply chain for our basic provisions like food, water, energy, and medical care.

The staggering number of Americans who (out of necessity) filed for unemployment benefits was yet another reminder of our lack of self-sufficiency. But how, you might be wondering, was this an example of that? After all, to control an unprecedented public health crisis, government authority forcefully closed businesses. The consequence was that many had to file for unemployment. Well, at the time the lockdowns began, an interesting statistic started circulating. That statistic showed that only around five percent of American workers had at least $10,000 of savings. In other words, at the start of the lockdowns, ninety-five percent of people were living paycheck to paycheck (or close to it) with very little emergency funds to live off in the event of a severe economic downturn like the kind we experienced.

Now, sure, you could easily shift the blame for our lack of financial resolve to outside systemic forces like the undeniably exploitive features of our modern capitalist system. But that argument only takes us so far because it removes the all-important factor of personal responsibility from the equation. The bottom line is if more of us had emphasized the importance of building a rainy-day fund, then we wouldn't have had to depend on the government so intensely when the proverbial "shit hit the fan."

Thankfully, that event delivered two revelations as they relate to self-sufficiency in the way of action. The first revelation is that becoming so is highly possible now in this age of ever-sophisticated channels of communication through the Internet. Today, we can literally pick up any sustainable skill such as starting a garden, canning food, or installing solar panels on our homes. No longer do we even need to go into the military or become an apprentice to acquire the very skills that we can now learn through our phones and computers. On this point, Sampson B., an art teacher from just outside Atlanta, Georgia, explained how starting a garden during the pandemic was as easy as watching a couple videos online:

> "As a city guy, prior to the pandemic, I knew nothing about gardening. Let alone how to start an organic garden. But when the pandemic hit, the latter was something that my partner and I were interested in starting. All it took was studying a couple YouTube™ videos to sort of get the basics. Now, I consider my partner and I to both be competent gardeners. In fact, we enjoyed such a great harvest in our first year that we were able to share our vegetables with all our neighbors. And mind you, this was done on only a quarter acre of land. [32]

My dear friend, Jamie Antoine, a motivational speaker, musician, and a black belt martial artist, also provides an inspiring example of someone who utilized his time spent in the lockdowns to become more self-sufficient in action. During that time, he became an expert gardener (Jamie grows some of the best hops around!) and took further steps to make his home more energy efficient. For as long as I have known him, Jamie has always emphasized the paramount importance of becoming self-sufficient in both thought and action because it leads to self-improvement and happiness. Jamie has always been fond of saying, "You have greatness in you." An inspirational phrase that I think we can all take to heart!

A second revelation that we all gleaned from our collective experience is that becoming self-sufficient is food for our souls. There is something inherently beneficial to our own spiritual growth when we learn to become self-sufficient. For one, we become more confident and able beings when we gain the skills needed for our own survival. The struggle in learning these new talents also makes us more self-resilient in the face of navigating obstacles along the way. We also find gratitude when we add new skills to our personal repertoire. Becoming self-sufficient will also inevitably deepen our relationship and sense of connection with Earth. Practices like farming, foraging, and building shelters have the effect of reverting us back into a state of communion with Earth and all her natural cycles.

Some years back, I spent an extremely hot summer (even by Southern Appalachian standards) working on a hemp farm in the North Carolina Mountains. Much of the work I did in the field was physically exhausting. Yet, despite enduring the hard labor and many pains in my body, I recall feeling strangely fulfilled while working there. I was learning how to farm, getting my hands dirty, and putting in an honest day's work. Furthermore, as the weeks went by my bond with the land and surrounding nature grew stronger. So much so that the farm began to feel like an extension of my being. As the cannabis plants began to mature, my connection to the land only heightened. While working on the farm I then began to truly understand what my old-time farmer neighbor, Rick, had meant when he once told me that he "feels closest to Christ" when he works the land behind his home. What I discovered in that summer on the farm is that learning self-sufficient skills not only makes us feel more confident, able, resilient, and fully connected beings, but it also brings us peace of mind.

Maddie S., an IT worker from Portland, Maine, expressed very similar feelings as I about learning a useful new skill. She explained how starting a greenhouse during the most recent pandemic brought her both a sense of purpose and connection that was missing in her life before:

> During the pandemic I was laid off from my job. Fortunately, I qualified for the expanded unemployment benefits. So, with my immediate financial stability somewhat assured, I decided to invest in building and starting a greenhouse. The project itself became something like a Zen art to me. There is just something so healing and pure about cultivating your own food to eat. I felt closer to Earth than I had at any time since I was a child. The funny thing is it really doesn't take much to grow your own food. But there are just so many forces out there trying to convince you that you need to depend on commercial agriculture. My message to everyone is that you, too, can produce a huge portion of what you consume. You must believe you can. That's all. [33]

In the end, becoming self-sufficient in action requires that we first become it in thought. To this point, G.I. Gurdjieff, the Greek Armenian spiritual teacher, said, "If you wish to get out of prison, the first thing you must do is realize that you are in prison. If you think you are free, you can't escape."[34]

If we continue to think we need the mass consumer machine to feed and supply us with our life necessities, then we will remain locked in our own prison of dependency believing we are free.

The Road to Self-Mastery

When we arrive at self-sufficiency in both thought and action, the road to self-mastery is open to be traveled on. Self-mastery is the realization of our fullest potential as incarnating souls taking birth in a physical body. In this metaphysical sense, we may be said to achieve self-mastery when our lives align with the highest qualities of the human spirit. These qualities include infinite compassion, inner faith in God or the One, the courage to keep on moving in the face of adversity, humility, simplicity in living — and not least of all, the wisdom gained from journeying to the mountaintop and back down to be shared with others.

The pursuit by all those on the spiritual path to cultivate each of these high qualities arises when we free our minds from cultural conditioning. In other words, to evolve in our consciousness we need to first become self-sufficient enough in our thoughts that we can naturally expand beyond our mind's limits. Without doing so we cannot hope to get very far on the path. If we allow our minds to be constantly inundated by the conditioned poisons of anger or greed, we will not become more compassionate beings. Likewise, if we constantly allow ourselves to be controlled by fear, we will never look within to find our refuge of courage. And if we embrace our culture's rampant narcissism, we will fail in our efforts to find humility and simplicity in our lives. Without finding humility and simplicity in our lives, how can we cultivate the necessary wisdom to be shared with others?

So, if we want to attain self-mastery as human beings, the first thing that we all must do is to train our minds (through practices like meditation) to become more one-pointed. This will help fortify our minds from the onslaught of toxicity that seeks to steer us into the abyss of negativity. But most important of all, we must each make the firm decision to embrace the unknown and push past our own sensual comforts. This is the essence of becoming self-sufficient in thought. Only when we are self-sufficient in thought are we ready to align our mind, body, and spirit with becoming self-sufficient in action.

Engaging in wholesome activities like, for example, growing our own food, cultivates all the inspiring qualities of self-mastery above. Providing for our own food through sustainable farming helps us overcome our fear of breaking free from mass consumer markets. It also builds our faith in Earth's natural cycles. Speaking of Earth, the cultivation of our gardens is a humbling experience that at once brings us in harmony with her marvelous simplicity. Whether we know it or not, when we share the fruits of our harvest with those in our communities we are engaging in an act of compassion. Through the ages, feeding those in need has always been regarded as a most holy act.

When the final story about the most recent pandemic is written, let it be known that that monumental event sparked a genuine desire within us to become self-sufficient in both thought and action. The road to self-mastery may now be a little more crowded than before.

Chapter Nine Key Takeaways

- There exist two kinds of self-sufficiency: self-sufficiency in thought and self-sufficiency in action.

- Self-sufficiency in thought means turning your mind to the truth within yourself and not to what is being propagandized on the outside. It means learning to think critically and forming your own thoughts about how to best navigate life and optimize opportunities for self-growth through spirited self-reflection.

- Self-sufficiency in action means engaging in activities with the intention of becoming independent through taking steps like growing your own food, collecting your own rainwater, and finding an alternative energy source to power your own home.

- Becoming self-sufficient in action provides many benefits for our spiritual path. For one, it brings great peace to our soul, teaches us to overcome adversity, helps us to cultivate greater gratitude in our daily lives, and makes us more confident and able beings.

- However, becoming truly self-sufficient in action requires that we first become so in thought.

- Unfortunately, the recent pandemic exposed in sometimes dramatic ways how far too many of us are not self-sufficient in either thought or action. Our adoption of extreme beliefs on both sides of the political spectrum in response to the crisis showed how too many of us are not yet self-sufficient in thought. And our extreme dependence on government entities during that event showed how we are not yet self-sufficient in action.

- However, a growing minority of people used the unique opportunities presented by the lockdowns to become more self-sufficient in both thought and action.

- In the end, self-sufficiency in both thought and action helps us achieve self-mastery.

Chapter Nine Meditation

Find a comfortable position seated either upright or in a cross-legged position. Now slowly close your eyes and turn your attention to your breath. Focus on allowing your mind to naturally expand. Let it expand beyond conceptual thought and into the realm of intuitive wisdom. Believe and know that your mind cannot be seduced by worldly pressures, temptations, or pleasures. For you are an incorruptible yogi and spiritual seeker who has risen beyond the temptations of this world. As you continue to inhale and exhale slow deep breaths, imagine your innermost being as a beacon of light breaking free through a prison cell of delusion, fear, and ignorance. Now, as the eternal witness, watch as your own inner light effortlessly races to expand past the walls of that prison, and into the countryside, through fertile green valleys, and up the tallest mountains. Take in this perspective that you have standing atop the rarified peaks.

Now, like an eagle, feel yourself soaring above your normal waking consciousness aware only of the natural spirit that knows no limits and no bounds. There is no one who can control your awareness because you are awareness itself running free. You are unfettered, independent in both thought and action and reliant on none other than Earth who provides you with your own daily sustenance through the sun and rain. Free in thought. Free in action. Self-sufficient. Fulfilled. Loved. Beyond birth. Beyond death. And beyond all the suffering of this world. Calm. Resolute in your purpose. Boundless in your compassion. All your worldly desires are extinguished. And all your sensual cravings now give way to the deathless spirit of intuitive wisdom. Intuitive wisdom is the path to your evolution as a conscious soul who has achieved self-mastery. Now open your eyes, take three slow deep breaths, and say these words out loud to yourself: "Here I am, and I have arrived. Thank you, Lord."

OM.

TEN
To Be and to Love

A Conversation with a Wise Friend

ONE day at the height of the lockdowns, I was sitting with Clay, a very dear and infinitely wise friend of mine. The two of us were basking in the spirit and talking about our connection to God. At some point during the discussion, Clay turned to me with a big smile on his face and said in a knowing tone that the point of life was "to be and to love." The meaning of life, he explained, was really that simple. According to my friend, there is never any need to over-intellectualize or philosophize about our existence. Rather, all we are called upon to do is to be and to love. Clay's words were such a revelation for me that when I got home that night, I pulled out my journal and tried to sincerely recall all the times in my life when I experienced the bliss of just being and loving.

I thought back to the innocence of my childhood, joyously playing capture the flag and basketball in the front yard with my friends without a care in the world. I thought of a poignant moment minutes before a high school track race when my father stood close behind me and showered me with unwavering love and support. I thought of the first day when I was finally off on my own in college and the overwhelming sense of freedom I felt. I thought of the day when Abbie, my beloved dog and best friend, first came into my life and the great joy it brought me. I then thought of meeting my kindred spirit, Rose, and feeling strangely certain that our meeting was more like a reunion of two souls over many lifetimes than the apparent introduction it was.

I thought of dancing at my first reggae show and feeling so connected to the music's sweet and soulful vibrations. I thought of numerous spirited hikes to the top of majestic peaks in both the Smoky and Rocky Mountains. I thought of my first meeting with Myrtle, the wise and godly Cherokee elder who would become a close friend and beloved teacher. I thought of a past trip to Maui, Hawaii and how that island's astounding beauty had opened my heart and awakened my spirit. I thought of the immense gratitude I felt for having the opportunity to perform live music for a period with two of my closest friends as crowds gathered around to hear our positive message. I also thought of the chance encounter that I had with a red-robed monk in the middle of a Nashville, Tennessee greenway and the extraordinary presence of compassion and equanimity that he radiated. Many other untold moments passed freely from my pen to paper as I reflected.

What was it about those moments, I asked myself, that had made them so memorable? Each of these moments brought me into the totality of being fully present with my heart wide open to the wonder of existence. In those precious instances, it is as if my mind stopped clinging to what the next sequence in my life would be. Instead of my mind being someplace else, I was just here, swimming in an ocean of pure awareness. These moments helped shape me to become who I really was. Though we all experience them, our acknowledgment of these type of profound and existential snapshots in time have become exceedingly rare.

This is because in our hyper-rationalist culture we tend to emphasize doing and acquiring over being and loving. However, learning to be and to love is one of the most important lessons that can be taken away from the time we spent in quarantine. Becoming who we are, in an age when all our vulnerabilities are laid bare, can feel especially daunting and heavy. But being and loving will always allow us to confront our deepest fears and anxieties with a certain quality of joy, lightness, and acceptance of what truly is. This way of relating to the world can help us all get on with our healing.

Obstructions to Being and Loving

To be means we must be here in this moment. Nowhere else. Not in the past. Not in the future. Just here in the present. But living in the Western world, our attention is almost totally directed on our past losses or traumas or on our future expectations. Usually, it is some combination of both. How different would our individual lives be if we could all be here? And how different would the whole world be if we could just be here? If we can't be present with one another, how can we even love one another? How can we be and love? For true love is expressed in the present moment when two or more souls come together in direct contact with the Highest. This is when we receive our spiritual nourishment. This is when we share in love.

During the most recent pandemic, many of us were left feeling so isolated and starving for affection that when the quarantine ended, we all re-emerged a little different than before. For a very brief period, many of us brought a heightened level of presence and awareness back into our interactions with others. I personally witnessed more people than ever before looking each other in the eyes when they talked. I saw more genuine displays of compassion between strangers than I had in a very long time. I also found myself immersed in conversations about higher consciousness with more people than I can ever recall having. Maybe it was the sheer delight from seeing others again face to face that temporarily improved our ability to be present. Or possibly, it was an expression of us being truly humbled by experiencing a collective period of hardship. I think both explanations somewhat explain why we grew in our awareness during that time. However, I intuitively feel that there is a third and even more convincing explanation for this. During the lockdowns, many of us were forced to sit, slow down, and focus inwardly on ourselves.

There is no doubt that being forced inward can cause immense discomfort at first. This discomfort is due to the waves of suffering that quickly rise to the surface within our minds. Just think for a moment about the great lengths we go to escape from our own pain. We distract ourselves with petty entertainment events, abuse alcohol and drugs, engage in promiscuous sex, whisper behind the backs of others, and try to consume our way into happiness. We only engage in these negative actions because we are trying to escape the hurt that results from living in a constant state of separation.

However, when we begin sitting with ourselves in ways that connect us with the living Spirit through practices like meditation, journaling, communing with nature, and chanting, we can't help but encounter the presence that is at the root of our very experience of being. This presence is always communicating in ways both subtle and not. And IT is responsible for why we breathe, why plants grow, why the sun shines, and why man and woman come together in sexual union to spawn new life. Meeting that presence has a way of making each one of us more present in our daily actions and injects our lives with meaning. Funny how that works. Another way to put it: the moment when we turn our hearts to God is when we can be and love. Here in the eternal now.

This higher state of awareness that I am trying to describe is what so many of us re-emerged with after the lockdowns. However, these soul revelations were unfortunately short-lived. Within a matter of months, there we were, right back at it again! Acquiring things that we didn't need, more addicted than ever before to social media and the convenience of online shopping, as well as being hyper-focused on the pursuit of money. In other words, we shifted back again from being to doing. Now, as it turns out, there is nothing wrong in principle with being a "doer." After all, just as Sri Krishna points out in the Bhagavad Gita, all beings in the wild (including humans) are moved to act. We must constantly be "doing" to carry out essential functions of life like procuring food, finding a mate, or caring for our children. But when our acts become hopelessly detached from the presence that is found when we are just "being" in moments of quiet reflection, prayer, or meditation, our acts are performed mindlessly and without awareness of why we act in the first place: to be love. Awareness of that love only comes when we act from the place where we are that love. But sadly, like we all experienced, all we wind up doing is erecting barriers to being and loving when our actions are performed without that kind of awareness.

The consequences of not acting from that state of loving awareness is obvious to see. Wars of aggression and the threat of a nuclear holocaust. The proliferation of gang warfare in our cities. Spiraling drug addiction and overdoses. The disturbing destruction of our beautiful planet by our own wasteful consumption habits. And the shameful exploitation of children and the poor. These are the social indicators of a society that has myopically followed the path of doing without ever stopping for a minute to consider the merits of the path of being. With the motors of the economy ground to a halt, the most recent pandemic provided us with a small window to seriously reconsider the path we were on. The question now before us is how do we break down the ego-driven barriers of complacency, fear, ignorance, and separation that were briefly challenged during the quarantine but then resurfaced once we returned to "normal"?

One answer to this question is for us to turn back to our religious faiths for guidance. But we must do this in a way that honors the mystical roots of each religion.

Back to Religion's Roots

Crisis situations like a pandemic demand a response from our religious traditions to help keep alive our faith. However, one thing we learned from the most recent pandemic is that an institutionalized hierarchy of powerful leaders and their followers no longer serve us. It may only exasperate our problems to be and to love even more. What we need, then, is a return to religion's roots. We need the inspiring wisdom of a Jesus or a Mohammad without the corrupt guidance of religious authorities. We need to touch the transcendent beauty of the Hindu or Jewish scriptures, firsthand, through one-pointed meditation. And we must see our own Buddha nature reflected in the life-giving rivers that flow effortlessly to the ocean.

At the roots of all the world's major religions are mystical traditions that emphasize the importance of our own direct intuitive experiences in connecting to God. In Christianity, these roots are discovered through emulating the lives of mystics like Saint Francis, Saint Teresa of Calcutta, and Thomas Merton, who were each a full embodiment of Christ's love. In Islam, the mystical tradition is expressed through

Sufi practices like the whirling dervishes (ecstatic dance) and through the inspired words of poet sages like Rumi and Hafiz. In Buddhism, it is found through Zen, a school of wisdom described by some as the "gateless gate," in which seekers arrive at their own enlightenment through persistent meditation (Zazen) and almost zero reliance on the word of scripture. In Hinduism, this mystical tradition is reflected in sacred texts like the Upanishads and the Bhagavad Gita, which both vividly describe the nature of Brahman, the supreme reality. It is also reflected in the practice of the many wandering Sadhus (holy men and women) who tirelessly search for an unfettered communion with God. And in Judaism, the mystical roots are manifested in Hasidism, a powerful and fascinating expression of that faith.

Aldous Huxley, the revered writer-sage, calls these common mystical ties in all religions the "perennial philosophy." This perennial philosophy, or whatever name we use to describe it, has the power to transform entire societies because it can change the hearts of all individuals from the inside out. More significantly, direct spiritual seeking has the power to heal division between groups of people and build peace among all God's children. Whenever we meditate or pray, we feel a deep kinship with all beings of Earth. It is this profound sense of interconnection that sparks monumental shifts in consciousness and breaks down barriers of separation. It is the illusion of separation that frustrates our attempts at peace in the first place. Anthropocentrism, racism, sexism, nationalism, and classism are all faces of a false reality that pictures the web of being as a collection of unrelated parts.

Our shared experience during the viral contagion made it abundantly clear that organized religion has failed us. At our time of need, many church leaders simply chose partisan politics and divisive rhetoric over compassion and love. At the height of that dramatic event, the Reverend David Wilson Rogers, a well-respected religious leader in the Christian community, wrote an op-ed piece to the Carlsbad Current-Argus that perfectly captured the churches' shortcomings:

> When it comes to COVID-19, the church has failed. As Christians, we have failed to follow biblical mandates, failed to honor and respect others, and failed to authentically embody the love of Jesus Christ. The root of the failure is idolatry. An idol in Scripture is anything that becomes the focus of worship, attention, and dedication which is not God. Although idolatry is nothing new in Christianity, the perverse distortions of the Christian faith that have permeated so much of our American culture are a huge part of the problem as to why Christianity has so miserably failed. Rather than trusting in Jesus Christ, far too many Christians have placed their ultimate trust in partisan politics. Worse yet, the reality of the pandemic was quickly weaponized by both extremes of the partisan ideological divide. Rather

than seeing the global pandemic as a public health crisis, it quickly was used to define partisan platforms, partisan belief systems, and fidelity to partisan ideals. [35]

Rogers continued to explain:

> As politicized anger and resentment over how the government was handling the pandemic (or not handling it as some would otherwise believe) Christians pushed the teachings about Christ aside in preference for doctrines, actions, and expressions that presumed to honor God, but actually only served to promote hate, anger, division, and sinful nationalism. No longer was the fight to protect humanity from the ravages of the pandemic, the fight turned into a bitterly angry tantrum over which political party was going to have the power, the control, and the ability to prove the other party to be wrong. Christianity failed because we sought power and control over surrender and service. Christianity failed because we chose to live in fear of a pandemic. Christianity has failed because people are more concerned about how the government, elected leaders, businesses, and institutions handled the controversy than we are about keeping people safe. Christianity failed the minute we embraced the lie that the pandemic was about partisan politics and not human health. [36]

Amen to Roger's words. But just because mainstream religion failed us doesn't mean that all hope is lost. Far from it. Though mainstream religion has clearly made a mockery of itself (at least here in the United States), returning to religion's roots is one way to heal the discord that is escalating throughout much of the world since the end of that difficult event. It is important to remember that the mystics of every faith have always been at odds with the leadership of institutionalized religion. Perhaps it is not all too surprising, then, that the Church spectacularly fell on its face during that time. For devoid of Christ's love, what is Christianity other than a hallow pillar of institutional authority? The same holds true for any religion. It is the mystics of every faith who have always injected living Spirit into religion. And it is the mystics of every faith who have always pointed the way for humanity to be and to love.

An Unbreakable Kind of Love

Many years back I had a mystical experience during meditation that still stands out in my mind. I described it in my first book, *The Hippie Revival*. I also shared it with thousands of listeners on the JeffMara Paranormal Podcast. The mystical experience (which really was a vision) was very brief but it left an indelible mark on my consciousness:

> *In my vision, I arrived at a place where I saw one large ring of people standing in puffy white clouds. The people were all smiling, laughing, and embracing one another. At first, I couldn't make out their faces. However, I felt as though I knew each person. As I walked over toward the ring, I began to make out the faces. I saw immediate family, current best friends, and my dog Abbie. I also saw three ex-girlfriends and my two closest friends from college. Going back further in time, I was astonished to find that my best friends from high school and childhood were there as well. Remarkably, the ring also included people with whom I had endured falling-outs with. For example, another ex-girlfriend stood in the ring smiling, as did my best friend from high school. He stood in the middle of the ring and extended his hand out to mine when I approached him. We then pulled each other in close for a hug. I took my place in the ring, and we all held hands and began to spin together in a circle. This was a dance of peace and harmony. The scene rushed over me with such positive vibrations that I felt waves of tears streaming down my face.* [37]

When I came out of this trance, I began to piece together the deeper meaning of this vision. I came to a simple revelation: life's highest purpose is to love. We are here to perfect its expression in human form. In this vision, I also saw that love is unconditional. It doesn't acknowledge tensions between close friends or loved ones. Rather, if any being touched your heart at any point in time, love shall prevail. Love is also eternal, as it transcends both time and space. In this vision, it was also clear to me that love knows nothing of separateness, only of oneness. I realized that the former emanates from the ego, and the latter from the depths of the soul. I also concluded that separateness arises from the ego's tendency to judge, label, and assign arbitrary values to being. This is the opposite case with our souls. On the soul plane, there is no judgment or separation. Only unconditional acceptance and love.

In the years and decades ahead, humanity is truly destined to realize what I only experienced in this fleeting vision: an unbreakable love that transcends all forms of separateness. This unconditional love is pure essence, pure being. It is true: the single greatest lesson that humanity can take away from any period of collective suffering is to be and to love.

Chapter Ten Key Takeaways

- The highest purpose of life is "to be and to love."

- The bliss from being and loving brings us into the totality of being fully present with our hearts wide open to the wonder of existence. In those precious instances, our minds stop clinging to what the next sequence in life should be.

- In our hyper-rationalist culture, we tend to emphasize doing and acquiring over being and loving.

- Learning to be and to love is one of the most important lessons that can be taken away from the most recent pandemic. Becoming who we are, in an age when all our vulnerabilities are laid bare, can feel especially daunting and heavy. But being and loving will always allow us to confront our deepest fears and anxieties with a certain quality of joy, lightness, and acceptance of what truly is. This way of relating to the world can help us all get on with our healing.

- When we begin sitting with ourselves in ways that connect us with the living Spirit through practices like meditation, journaling, communing with nature, and chanting, we can't help but encounter the "presence" — the underlying energy or intelligence that is at the root of the very experience of being. This presence is always communicating in ways both subtle and not. Meeting that presence has a way of making each one of us more present in our daily actions and injects our lives with meaning.

- We re-emerged with a higher state of consciousness after the lockdowns. However, it was unfortunately short-lived as we shifted back again from being to doing.

- The consequences of not acting from that state of awareness are obvious to see. Wars of aggression and the threat of a nuclear holocaust. The proliferation of gang warfare in our cities. Spiraling drug addiction rates and overdoses. The disturbing destruction of our beautiful planet by our own wasteful consumption. And the shameful exploitation of children and the poor. These are the social indicators of a society that has myopically followed the path of doing without ever stopping for a minute to consider the merits of the path of being.

- The question before us now is how to break down the ego-driven barriers of complacency, fear, ignorance, and separation that were briefly challenged during the most recent pandemic but then quickly resurfaced once we returned to "normal."

- Crisis situations like a pandemic demand a response from our religious traditions to help keep alive our faith.

- The recent pandemic made it abundantly clear that organized religion has failed us. At people's time of desperate need, many church leaders chose partisan politics and divisiveness over compassion and love.

- Returning to religion's roots (mysticism) is one way to heal the discord that is escalating throughout much of the world since the end of the last pandemic.

- The single greatest lesson that we can take away from the most recent pandemic is to be and to love.

Chapter Ten Meditation

Find a comfortable position seated either upright or with legs crossed. Now close your eyes and tune into your breath. Breathe in and breathe out. As you inhale and exhale, let all thoughts and worries fall from your mind. Now, silently offer any regrets from the past or any anxieties over the future as sacrificial offerings to a deity, guru, or holy figure such as Buddha, Christ, or Shiva. As you make your offer, focus your attention on your third eye (the sacred chakra point between your two eyebrows) and repeat these words to yourself: "I am a point of sacrificial fire, held within the fiery will of God." Keep on repeating this mantra until your mind begins to grow quieter. As your mind quiets, bring your focus to the quality of being. Notice the feelings of peace, serenity, and stillness that flood your mind, body, and soul as you embrace the act of being. You are the master over your own mind. You are the master of your own universe. Now, let your consciousness expand as you allow yourself the liberty to fully explore the depths of your soul. You are boundless like the ocean. Resolute like a mountain. And as free as a leaf blowing in the wind. Do you feel now what it means to really be? As you continue centering yourself, try to open your heart as you try and recall a being who captures the essence of love. What are the characteristics of this being? Infinite compassion? Loving kindness? Uncompromising faith and humility? In what ways can you feel their overflowing love? Open yourself to that love. Now, take a moment and acknowledge the sheer power of just being and loving. You are that.

Now re-open your eyes and rest in the stillness. That is your birthright as an incarnating soul in a physical body — to rest in that sacred space beyond time. Remember, there is no past. There is no future. There is only now. There is only here. Absolute being. Pure unconditional love. That is what you are. To be and to love.

OM.

Bibliography

1. Vivekananda, Swami. Essay. In *The Complete Works of Swami Vivekananda*, 451. New York, NY: Discovery Publisher, 2019.

2. Rivers, Forrest, and Jason P. Interview with Jason P. Personal, November 13, 2021.

3. Rivers, Forrest, and Alex C. Interview with Alex C. Personal, October 16, 2021.

4. Rivers, Forrest, and Erica B. Interview with Erica B. Personal, October 30, 2021.

5. Rivers, Forrest, and Lisa K. Interview with Lisa K. Personal, March 23, 2022.

6. Rivers, Forrest, and Paul G. Interview with Paul G. Personal, March 14, 2022.

7. Rivers, Forrest, and Brett U. Interview with Brett U. Personal, December 14, 2021.

8. Rivers, Forrest, and Leila Hancock. Interview with Leila Hancock. Personal, June 22, 2022.

9. Rivers, Forrest, and Dylan F. Interview with Dylan F. Personal, May 6, 2022.

10. Ibid.

11. Rivers, Forrest, and Nick P. Interview with Nick P. Personal, December 7, 2021.

12. Rivers, Forrest, and Elijah Dicks. Interview with Elijah Dicks. Personal, December 7, 2021.

13. Rivers, Forrest, and Cassandra S. Interview with Cassandra S. Personal, December 3, 2021.

14. Dass, Ram. In *Paths to God: Living the Bhagavad Gita*, 2–3. New York, NY: Three Rivers, 2006.

15. Groves, Bill. "The Spirituality of Surrender." Speech, August 7, 2022.

16. Rivers, Forrest, and Chris G. Interview with Chris G. Personal, September 20, 2022.

17. Ibid.

18. Rivers, Forrest, and Sandy D. Interview with Sandy D. Personal, October 2, 2022.

19. Ibid.

20. Rivers, Forrest, and Raphael C. Interview with Raphael C. Personal, January 8, 2022.

21. Ibid.

22. Reif, Max. "6 Weeks of Shelter-in-Place: Personally, and Socially Where Is This Leading?" The Mindful Word, April 29, 2020. https://www.themindfulword.org/.

23. Rivers, Forrest, and Kevin S. Interview with Kevin S. Personal, July 2, 2022.

24. Ibid.

25. Rivers, Forrest, and Taylor R. Interview with Taylor R. Personal, July 17, 2022.

26. Rivers, Forrest, and Carol. Email exchange with Carol. Personal, May 17, 2022.

27. Steel Pulse. *Rollerskates*. CD. *Rastanthology*, 1984.

28. Rivers, Forrest, and Austin S. Interview with Austin S. Personal, November 13, 2021.

29. Rivers, Forrest, and Diana P. Interview with Diana P. Personal, February 18, 2022.

30. Rivers, Forrest, and Dave. Dave's Story. Personal, n.d.

31. Gaskin, Stephen. Essay. In *This Season's People: A Book of Spiritual Teachings*, 1st ed., 119. Summertown, TN: Book Pub. Co., 1976.

32. Rivers, Forrest, and Sampson B. Interview with Sampson B. Personal, August 5, 2022.

33. Rivers, Forrest, and Maddie S. Interview with Maddie S. Personal, August 8, 2022.

34. Gurdjieff, Georges Ivanovitch. In *Beelzebub's Tales to His Grandson: All and Everything*, 112. London: Arkana, 2000.

35. Rogers, Rev. David Wilson. "The Church Has Failed in COVID-19 Pandemic." *Carlsbad Current Argus*. November 13, 2021. https://www.currentargus.com/news/.

36. Ibid.

37. Rivers, Forrest. Essay. In *The Hippie Revival and Collected Writings*, 34. Scotts Valley, CA: CreateSpace, 2016.

Forrest Rivers

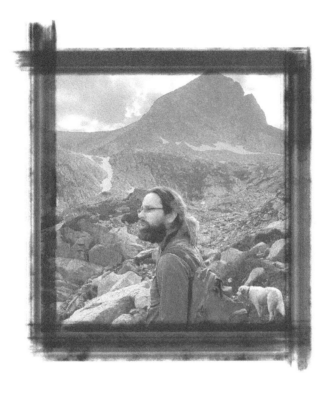

FORREST RIVERS is a seeker and lover of Earth who enjoys hiking with his dog, Abbie. He is the author of *The Hippie Revival and Collected Writings*, and a collection of short stories titled *Beyond the Void: Parables for a Waking World*. You can reach Forrest through his website, forrestrivers.com, and follow him on Facebook or through his YouTube™ channel, "Mystic Soul Revival with Forrest Rivers."

Milton Keynes UK
Ingram Content Group UK Ltd.
UKHW041539121024
449426UK00005B/372